D1721121

AYAHUASCA

Sacred Plant Medicine of the Amazon Jungle

By
Naomi Harper

© Copyright 2019 by Naomi Harper - All rights reserved.

This book is provided with the sole purpose of providing relevant information on a specific topic for which every reasonable effort has been made to ensure that it is both accurate and reasonable. Nevertheless, by purchasing this book you consent to the fact that the author, as well as the publisher, are in no way experts on the topics contained herein, regardless of any claims as such that may be made within. As such, any suggestions or recommendations that are made within are done so purely for entertainment value. It is recommended that you always consult a professional prior to undertaking any of the advice or techniques discussed within.

This is a legally binding declaration that is considered both valid and fair by both the Committee of Publishers Association and the American Bar Association and should be considered as legally binding within the United States.

The reproduction, transmission, and duplication of any of the content found herein, including any specific or extended information will be done as an illegal act regardless of the end form the information ultimately takes. This includes copied versions of the work both physical, digital and audio unless express consent of the Publisher is provided beforehand. Any additional rights reserved.

Furthermore, the information that can be found within the pages described forthwith shall be considered both accurate and truthful when it comes to freely available information and general consent. As such, any use, correct or incorrect, of the provided information will render the Publisher free of responsibility as to the actions taken outside of their direct purview. Regardless, there are zero scenarios where the original author or the Publisher can be deemed liable in any fashion for any damages or hardships that may result from any of the information discussed within.

Finally, any of the content found within is ultimately intended for entertainment purposes and should be thought of and acted on as such. Due to its inherently ephemeral nature nothing discussed within should be taken as an assurance of quality, even when the words and deeds described herein indicated otherwise. Trademarks and copyrights mentioned within are done for informational purposes in line with fair use and should not be seen as an endorsement from the copyright or trademark holder.

Disclaimer

This book is intended for informational purposes only. People wishing to drink Ayahuasca should consult their medical doctors before engaging with this medicine. The use, possession, and trafficking of Ayahuasca are illegal in many countries, and the author doesn't condone the breaking of the laws of any country.

TABLE OF CONTENTS

Introduction.. 1

Chapter 1 *Origin Story, Cultural And Mythic Archetypes*........................... 2

Chapter 2 *The Role Of The Shaman*... 13

Chapter 3 *Chemical Effects On The Body And The Brain* 23

Chapter 4 *Preparation* 35

Chapter 5 *The Experience* 47

Chapter 6 *Long-Term Effects* 58

Conclusion 68

Description...69

INTRODUCTION

Congratulations on purchasing *Ayahuasca: Sacred Plant Medicine of the Amazon Jungle,* and thank you for doing so.

The following chapters will discuss the sacred hallucinogenic tea known as ayahuasca, as well as the specifics of the culture and practices surrounding it. First, we will delve into the mythic origin of the plant, and the stories that are told about its origins—as well as the sacred animals associated with it. We will also explore the cultural significance of the tea and the ceremonies surrounding it to everyday life in the people of the Amazon.

Then, we will define and explore the role of the shaman as the facilitator of the experience, and then we will delve into the neurobiological effects of the medicine. Once we have explored the chemistry of the medicine, we will then define the extensive preparation rituals and regimens prescribed prior to the experience.

After this, the book will delve into the various aspects of the experience itself, as well as the categories of journey one may undergo under the influence of the medicine. Finally, we will learn about the importance of after-care and integration to having a successful long-term prognosis, as well as the ailments ayahuasca has been known to alleviate or outright cure (including but not limited to addiction, depression, and PTSD).

There are plenty of books on this subject on the market, thanks again for choosing this one! Every effort was made to ensure it is full of as much useful information as possible, please enjoy!

CHAPTER 1

Origin Story, Cultural And Mythic Archetypes

In the Stories

According to the stories, the first humans came down from the sky in a serpent canoe, and the Sun Father promised to bequeath them a supernatural drink that would allow them to connect with the powers of the sky and the heavens. The men went to a place called "The House of Waters" in order to try and create this supernatural drink. While they were toiling away and attempting to create it, the first woman wandered into the forest; she was pregnant and entered the jungle in order to give birth. Her child was a boy who radiated golden light; after he was born, she rubbed him down with sacred leaves. Her child was the sacred ayahuasca vine.

When she returned, each of the men who had been trying to create the sacred drink cut off a piece of his body; each of these pieces became a part of that man's sacred lineage.

There are many cultures in the upper Amazon that utilize this sacred medicine, and thus there are many stories about how the medicine came to the people. These origin stories are intricately and intimately related to the cultures from which they grew, and can provide an understanding of their perspective and worldview, especially in relation to the sacred plants.

In other versions of this story, the first people came down from the sky from the Milky Way in a serpent canoe. They came from the Milky Way, and in their canoe, they brought three sacred plants: caapi (ayahuasca), coca, and cassava. The indigenous people largely believed the ayahuasca vine to be the Sun's gift to humankind, and a container for his light. The ayahuasca vine was also a gift showing them the right way to live and the right way to speak.

Another Tukano tale holds that a woman was impregnated through her eye by the Sun God and that her child was born in a flash of light. The woman cut the umbilical cord and began to rub her child's body with magical herbs, shaping it into the sacred ayahuasca vine, known to them as Caapi. Cappi became known as an old man who guarded the secrets and power of the ayahuasca vine. To these people, sex is a visionary and hallucinogenic experience in which the men "drown" in visions. Thus, Cappi is not only the guardian of the ayahuasca vine, but also of the sexual potency of men, the mythological source of their semen, and the source of the visions they experience during intercourse.

From a different indigenous tribe, they tell of Yagé Woman, yage being another indigenous word for ayahuasca. At the beginning of time, when the serpent canoe was moving up the rivers in order to settle humankind.

When the canoe landed at the House of Waters, Yagé Woman appeared. In front of the village center, she gave birth. She took the leaves of a plant and cleaned off both herself and her child. After she had given birth, the umbilical cord became the ayahuasca vine, and the leaves became an essential ingredient in the sacred brew.

Still, other stories from other tribes tell that the medicine was conceived between the Sun Father and his daughter, who gave birth to the vine. Yet more tell that the sacred knowledge was gifted to them from the mysterious and secret underwater realm, or was created from a giant serpent's tail that joined earth and heaven.

In one tale concerning the sacred brew, there was a woman named Kamaisani. This woman lived off by herself, but her brother sent his children to her to get some chichi, which is a kind of alcoholic drink. Being stingy, Kamaisani sent them away. When his children returned, Kamaisani's brother had them gather caapi. The brother and his children chewed the vine and ascended into the sky, and did not invite his sister because she had been stingy. However, Kamaisani found out and chewed caapi to also join them in the heart of the sky. Because of her stinginess, they did not let her live with them; thus, she had to go live in another part of the sky away from all the other stars.

The myths that describe a woman conceiving the ayahuasca vine by being impregnated by the Sun God can be understood as an alchemical metaphor, allowing a human to join with the heavenly light. Whether the medicine's origin story is about the Sun God impregnating a woman, or a serpent that joins heaven and earth, or a gift from the secret underwater world, they all share one thing in common. All of these stories are ways of describing how ordinary human consciousness can access the divine through the visionary medicine of ayahuasca.

Nearly all of the myths tell of how the sacred ayahuasca vine or child was wiped off with special herbs or leaves. The ayahuasca brew cannot be made from the ayahuasca vine alone. Rather, it must be combined with other plants and cooked down. This is reflected in the myths, where in some cases the child is cleaned or even "shaped" with special herbs or leaves. The combination of these different plants creates the psychoactive elements of the brew.

Cultures around the world don't just use myths to tell stories around the fire. The myths help people understand something fundamental about the world and the way in which it works, and the way in which they relate to it. When you learn the myths of the culture you are also learning about the lens through which they view the world. Knowing that these cultures view the ayahuasca vine as something given from the divine and that the vine has the power to launch people "into the eye of the sky," it tells you something about not only the ways in which they use the medicine but also the medicine itself.

Each cultural group in the Amazon has its own variations on the origin myth of the ayahuasca vine. Subtly or drastically different myths are indicative of how each culture has a different relationship to the vine and uses it in different ways. The myths of any culture grow naturally out of the ecology of the line in which they are based. Therefore, each different ecological area will have naturally occurring variations in there ceremonial methods and tools.

In the Culture

Ancient History of the Sacrament

There is no exact timeline as to when ayahuasca was discovered. This information is unknowable due to the fact that it occurred several thousands of years ago, and no written records exist from that time. However, there is a large amount of indirect archaeological evidence that points to the plant's antiquity. There have been discoveries of anthropomorphic figurines, pottery vessels, trays and tubes for snuffing, etc. which all point to a well-seated use of hallucinogenic herbs and plants at least four thousand years ago.

While it is very clear that the ancient Amazonians were using hallucinogenic plants of many varieties (such as coca, tobacco, and psychoactive snuffs), the aforementioned archaeological evidence does not point to ayahuasca use specifically. However, despite the fact that there is no concrete evidence, these ancient Amazonian cultures had a complex understanding of the psychopharmacology of many different kinds and combinations of plants. It would then be entirely within the realm of possibility that they also knew of ayahuasca.

This lack of clear and specific evidence attesting to the medicine's first conception and use has been the bane of many a Western scientist and anthropologist, due to the modern preoccupation and fascination that academia has fixed on this medicine since at least the 1960s. The reason that academics are so flustered is the fact that that ayahuasca brew does not contain only one plant. It is a combination of two plants—neither of which is particularly psychoactive on their own. The means through which someone combined them, whether through accident or experimentation, is a mystery. Someone had to be the first one to combine the two plants to create the hallucinogenic tea. Scientists have spent much effort attempting to clarify who this person was and where they lived, but there has been little in the way of evidence to help them in their task.

The only clear fact is that wherever the medicine originated, the protocols for gathering, preparing, cooking, and administering the plant spread throughout the entire upper Amazon well before the first Westerners ever made their way to South America.

Plants as Teachers

While the historical origin of the medicine is lost to time, the mythic origin provides quite a few explanations as to the origin of the medicine. While many cultures have a story describing the gifting of ayahuasca to the people by the Sun God or otherworldly beings, the indigenous people of Peru have a slightly different perspective.

To the indigenous people of Peru, the way that humans came to have ayahuasca was not through gifting from heavenly or otherworldly beings. Rather, they attained the knowledge directly from the plants themselves. How did they do this? They say that they gained this knowledge directly from the plants themselves.

There are many ways in which this knowledge is revealed. A shaman may be under the influence of a particular plant sacrament and receive insight. This insight can come from the plant currently in their system, or as a conversation from a plant in their proximity. In this conversation with the plant, it is revealed to the shaman what plant must be gathered, how it must be prepared, the protocols for its use, and what need in the community the plant's use will serve. There are stories of shamans wandering off into the jungle without a word, and returning months or years later with advanced herbal knowledge learned directly from the spirits of the jungle. Occasionally plant medicine lore is also revealed through visions or dreams sent from the plant teachers.

However the information is attained, one thing is very clear. The people of the upper Amazon have a fundamentally different understanding of mind and consciousness than Westerners. To the people of the Amazon, plants are not only sentient beings, but they are also beings that have intention, desire, and will. These beings deliberately seek to create relationships with human beings and to pass on wisdom. When you consider a worldview in which plants are sentient, communicative entities, something as simple as a walk through the jungle takes on a very different kind of significance.

Indigenous Cosmology

The indigenous people of the Amazon have a fundamentally different relationship to the plants around them. Understanding the above, one can begin to understand how this small slice of information is a window to a completely different perspective for understanding the world. This is a cosmology in which the spiritual world is immanent, plants have consciousness, both light and dark magic are widespread, and these powers can be accessed through the ceremonial brewing and ingestion of various combinations of sacred herbs.

People who live in these cultures are constantly surrounded by the sacred. There are always spirits, energies, and peoples that are seeking to influence an individual. The ability of one to avoid these influences or to take on beneficial influences is attributed as a source of social standing and influence as well as personal success. If negative events or bad luck begin to plague a person, their spiritual system compels them to look to the realm of the spirits for an answer.

Ayahuasca is a critical tool that helps shamans gain access to information that is typically hidden from the layman's eyes. With the help of this plant, the shaman can peer into the spirit world and see the unseen to identify the source of the trouble.

There are many occasions that would prompt a shaman to use ayahuasca to peer into the spirit world. These include straightforward cases of sickness and wounds, to more complicated social strife, to environmental phenomena such as earthquakes or droughts. All of these things have a root cause in the spirit world, and ayahuasca helps the shaman to discover what those reasons are.

This is a stark contrast to the purely materialistic and consumer-minded nature of Western culture. The Western mindset would have one believe that the world stops and ends at what you can see, touch, hear, smell, and taste. To many hardline Western materialists, not only are spirits nonexistent, but those who believe in them are delusional. Further, this divide in cosmology is what has led to the plundering of the Amazon for its natural resources, such as lumber and oil. The land is staunchly defended by people who believe the jungle is full of sentient and sacred entities, while it is attacked by those who believe neither in non-human sentience nor sacredness.

In the Spirit World

There are beings and entities that move through the world of the spirits. Some of those entities and spirits are named and have become intimately linked with the ceremonies and protocols of the ayahuasca shaman. Among those entities are the spirits of the snake, jaguar, eagle, and condor. Each of these four animals has a unique archetypal energy and arrives for different reasons. Each may be invoked during the ceremony for different purposes, depending on the needs of the moment.

Snake

Serpents are extremely prevalent in the mythos of the upper Amazon. It was a serpent canoe that brought the people to the Earth, and in some stories, a sacred serpent's tail turned into the ayahuasca plant. In part, this is likely because of the profusion of snakes in the local ecology; it would make sense that they would occupy a place of mythic significance. If encountered from a place of trust and surrender, the snake is a benevolent entity to help you along your healing path. If encountered with resistance and fear, the snake can easily become a demonic specter that haunts the visions of those to ingest the medicine. If one has an exposure to Christian theology and teachings, then the snakes may also occupy this archetype during that person's experience.

Some people journeying on the medicine actually experience the spirit of ayahuasca appearing to them as a giant serpent. The medicine itself may be personified through the snake. The snake appears in many forms, and many ways. People have reported vomiting up many thousand small, black snakes. Others have reported being invited to ride on the back of a snake. Still others become the snake and feel themselves slithering along the ground as if they were a serpent. While still valid, all of these are considered inferior to the primary snake experience. This experience involves being swallowed whole.

The snake is not merely the spirit of the plant, but also the spirit of the cosmos, the primordial information that humans are seeking to tap into. It is not only the Caapi that launched Kamaisani into the "eye of the sky"—it is the eye of the sky itself. Once one has been swallowed into the gullet of the cosmic serpent, it is believed that one has been initiated and accepted by the medicine. Now that the person has been taken into the spirit of the medicine, their healing can begin.

The snake itself is representative across many cultures (including those of the upper Amazon) of both transformation and rebirth. Whether one thinks of the alchemical snake biting its own tail (ouroboros), or the cosmic serpent, the primary happening is transmutation. When the snake sheds its skin, it looks as if it is emerging from the amniotic sack. It has the ability to shed what is old and dead and emerge refreshed and renewed. This is one reason why it is such a powerful healing spirit in conjunction with ayahuasca.

One is rarely if ever, swallowed by the serpent while they still fight and resist. Learning to humble oneself and surrender is vital in order to be accepted by this spirit. Only once someone has learned to metaphorically kneel before spirit and accept their own fallibility as a human will they be accepted into the serpent's maw.

For the shaman who is under the influence of ayahuasca, there is another added dimension to the snake imagery. Shamans have the ability to "suck" illness and troubles out of the body of their patients. When the illness emerges, to the shaman's vision, it may appear as if black snakes are being pulled from the body. To the patient under the influence of ayahuasca, if they are purging, they may see their own vomit as many black snakes emerging from their mouths. For the shaman's apprentice, who is still learning the territory of the altered state, the vision of the snakes has yet more layers of meaning.

At the beginning of their training, the initiate may see large masses of curling snakes. The curling mass of snakes represents the curling masses of the ayahuasca vine, as well as nature as a whole. Its wild, unwieldy tangles and size stand for the task ahead of the initiate, as well as for the tangles within the initiate's own mind. Once the initiate has begun to

7

learn how to work with altered states of consciousness, the tangles begin to sort themselves out. And once the initiate has mastered the ayahuasca vine, it is believed that they also have mastered nature itself and can walk impervious where other people would find danger.

The Conibo-Shipibo people believe that once an apprentice has been initiated, they will acquire giant spirit-serpents which will defend them from the black arts of sorcerers. These spirit-serpent helpers help the shamans in all manner of tasks, from fending off enemy shamans to assisting in the retrieval of lost parts of the soul. Attaining these spirit-helpers is a mark that one has begun to master the skills necessary to operate as a full shaman.

Snakes and serpents are woven intricately throughout the stories and consciousness of the people of both Mesoamerica and South America. The pre-Incan society known as the Chavín heavily featured snake iconography in all of their art. The secrets of their serpent-worship have been lost to time. In Mesoamerica, Quetzalcoatl is regarded as the savior of humankind. Although Quetzalcoatl appears sometimes as a man, he also appears as a flying rainbow serpent. This serpent not only made key contributions to the creation of humankind and their education and learning, but he was also able to act as a bridge of connection between the realms of the Earth and the Sky. This linking of the realms of the transcendent to the earthly, and providing teachings are closely related to the ways snake spirits operate in relation to ayahuasca.

Snakes have many roles in the ayahuasca ceremony. They can be the physical embodiment of an illness that a shaman pulls from the body. They can be tangled masses which represent the tangles within one's own mind. Snakes may appear as guides to assist with the work of the shaman. Most profoundly and powerfully, snakes may act as a gateway to the primordial, swallowing the initiate whole and initiating them into the path of their own healing. There is no one single way the snake appears during the ceremony and the experience of it is highly individuated and based on circumstance.

Jaguar

These cats are powerful entities, both in the realm of the physical and in the realm of the spirit. While the spirit of the snake is intimately linked with the spirit of ayahuasca, one could say the jaguar is more intimately connected to the spirit of the shaman. Just because it is linked with humans, though, does not bespeak a lack of power.

In many of the languages of the upper Amazon, the word for "shaman" and the word for "jaguar" are one and the same. Why is this so? It is commonly believed that shamans have the power to shapeshift into a jaguar, either physically or in spirit-form. The body of the shaman is able to house both spirits, and from this spirit, the shaman draws his power.

Jaguars are largely associated with shape-shifting, both in the literal sense as well as in the transformative sense. There is a slight differentiation between the properties of the regular jaguar spirit and that of the black jaguar spirit. The black jaguar is far rarer and has an additional layer of symbolism. It is revered as a gatekeeper to the realms of time.

While there is a clear spiritual dimension to the mythos of the jaguar, physical jaguars also have a link to the ayahuasca vine. It has been well-recorded that jaguars in the wild will deliberately seek out the sacred vine. Once they have located the vine, they will proceed to chew on it and ingest parts of the plant. Once they have ingested the plant, these jaguars proceed to behave in an entranced and delirious state, obviously having some kind of visionary or ecstatic experience. On a purely functional level, the ayahuasca vine is a powerful purgative and helps to cleanse the cat's stomach and digestive tract of parasites and other problems. The indigenous people of the upper Amazon also speculate that jaguars ingest the vine in order to heighten their hunting skills. A common effect noted in ayahuasca ceremonies is a heightening of the five senses of sight, smell, hearing, touch, and taste.

While in the ceremony, shamans would sometimes call on the spirit of the jaguar to guard the entrance to the maloca or central hut. This kept the ceremony's participants safe and kept away malevolent or trickster spirits. Jaguars can be called upon to take a protective role and as guardians of the doorway. Depending on the needs of the ceremony, the shaman may choose to call the typical jaguar, or its specialized cousin, the black jaguar.

In the stories of the indigenous peoples, the daytime noon sun was equated with the eagle and life-giving brilliance. At night the sun disappeared over the edge of the world; where it went was shrouded in mystery. Jaguars move through the night, the realm of the unknown. They do so with confidence and strength, with keen vision and great stealth. They are masters of the dark world. Thus, the hidden nighttime sun became known as the "jaguar sun."

Jaguars prefer to live in places that are close to sources of fresh water; water, as a reminder, commonly represents the human emotional body and subconscious. These watery places often include canyons or caves. The places where the earth opens are commonly believed to be entrances to the underworld. Jaguars are equated with the place below the earth where the daytime sun journeys at night. He is the ruler of the underworld and is believed to also be the force that lives inside of mountains, below the ground. It is this force that gives the mountains their explosive and volcanic father. Jaguar is considered not only to be an "Earth Father," but also King of the Animals

Among the Mesoamericans, jaguars were considered gods by the Aztec, Maya, Inca, and Olmec people. All of these people carved jaguar images into their pots, cookware, into their thrones, and into effigies in their temples. These images existed everywhere from the sacred to the profane.

Their images were woven into the funeral shrouds and shawls of the Chavín. Some Amazonian tribes ceremonially drank the blood of the jaguar, ate the heart of the jaguar, and wore the skin of the jaguar. The belief existed that not only could shamans turn into jaguars, but that jaguars could turn into humans. They are regarded as incredibly powerful spirits. In northwestern Columbia, the Desana people regarded the jaguar as the living manifestation of the sun's energy. In Bolivia, those who were most highly considered for the role of the shaman were those who had survived an attack by a jaguar. The Tucano people believed that the jaguar's roar foretold rain. In Mexico, the people parade through the streets wearing spotted regalia and jaguar masks in order to ask the jaguar god for rain and an abundant harvest.

There is a link between the jaguar's fiery power that lives beneath the earth, and with the water that denotes the human emotional subconscious. When it appears during the ceremony, it is experienced as the energy of life in its most raw and primal form. It is often experienced as a "cat of fire," and there is sometimes a transfer of energy between the patient and the spirit of the jaguar.

When jaguar appears in a ceremony, the experience tends to be an interactive one. They transfer energy to the patient, or oftentimes the patient finds themselves riding on the back of the jaguar. Patients may experience visits to the underworld while accompanied by this spirit, due to its links with the realms beneath the Earth. Someone may find themselves engaging in a process of life review, or of noticing patterns of behavior that they may not have previously noticed. The key eyesight of the jaguar may allow the patient to temporarily have the ability to see patterns amidst chaos. That night vision, coupled with the jaguar's raw power, also represents moving without fear through the darkness. This may be the darkness of the world or the darkness of one's own traumas and shadows.

Condor and Eagle

There is an ancient prophecy regarding the spirits of the condor and the eagle.

This prophecy describes how humanity's destiny would split down two roads, the road of the eagle, and the road of the condor. The road of the condor is the path of intuition, the heart, and of feminine energy. The eagle's road, on the other hand, is the path of the industrial, the mind, and masculine energy. In this prophecy, it is stated that in the 1490s (the year of Columbus's expedition to the Americas), a 500-year period would begin. During this period, the eagle people would become so powerful that they would nearly drive the condor people to extinction.

When one looks at the prophecy metaphorically, they could see how the USA is represented by the eagle, and how they are the stewards of Western values. The condor, on the other hand, represents the indigenous people who have kept their traditions alive throughout the ages, despite encroachment and oppression. On a more literal level, one could see this metaphor play out in the near-extinction of the California condor.

The second half of this prophecy states that there would be an opportunity for the eagle and the condor people to finally come together, and fly together. Metaphorically, this would mean a healing between the Western peoples and the indigenous peoples, a higher level of consciousness for humankind, and the sharing of knowledge. This prophecy perhaps an underlying reason why so many Westerners are now seeking ayahuasca treatment in the upper Amazon, and are seeking greater and more authentic connection with the Earth.

These birds also hold a vital place in the cosmology of many indigenous South American people. There is a three-way division of the cosmos. The lower or underworld is associated with the jaguar. This current level of reality is associated with the snake. The upper world, the realm of the gods, is associated with the eagle and condor.

These birds represent the sovereignty of the sky and the light of the sun, being called divine messengers. Out of all creatures, they exist closest to the sky and the heavens. Existing in this highest realm, closest to the gods, they represent the heights of spiritual attainment and the highest embodiment of humankind's values. Ascending as they do between the earth and the sky, they carry the messages of the gods to humankind. Their heavenly perspective also represents grand and far-seeing vision, and the ability to see reality for what it is and understand situations and circumstances in their totality.

In ceremonies, shamans may transform into birds—most commonly, the condor and the eagle. Aside from the jaguar, birds are the most common alter-ego of the shaman. The bird-form allows the shaman to ascend to the heavens and converse with the gods, gaining knowledge that they can use to help their patients and their people. They attain the ability to bridge the realms of heaven and the realms of earth from the eagle and condor.

It is not only the shaman that is able to take on the form of a bird, however. It is a common belief among the people of the upper Amazon that the inner form of the human soul is that of a bird. They believe that, at the time of death, the soul is released from the body in the form of a bird. The soul bird then flies to a predetermined destination. In some cultures, they believe that if the person has been good, they will go up to the sky and dwell with the gods. There is no one definitive myth that states where people who have lived poorly end up.

Similarly, in ceremony, someone's consciousness may also ascend to the sky with help from the condor, eagle, or other bird. The person may feel as if they are riding on the back of the eagle or condor, or maybe they have sprouted the wings of those birds from their bodies. Once they have ascended to the heavens, the experiences in these realms typically involve interacting with star-beings or deities. The exact details of the interactions are hugely varied depending on the individual, but the vehicle is consistent.

Cosmologically speaking, these three animals each serve a distinct function. The Cosmic Serpent represents all that is contained within this reality and its wisdom. The Jaguar represents the strength and vitality of life. The Condor and Eagle represent the love and light of the divine. All three are vital to the use of the other. Wisdom, when not lit with love and applicable to everyday life, is useless. Power devoid of love is dangerous. When wisdom, strength, and love come together, true change is made, and true healing is done.

CHAPTER 2
The Role Of The Shaman

The shaman is the central figure to the ayahuasca experience. Someone can take the medicine, but without the shaman, they will simply drift through the experience like a boat lost at sea. The shaman guides the experience as if steering a boat, creating a protected space in which people may confront their trauma and engage in deep healing. This chapter will delve into the life of the shaman—how they are chosen, their initiation process, and the training they receive. Secondly, this chapter will explore the tools and techniques that shamans employ both within and outside of ceremonial space and the kinds of functions they serve. Finally, this chapter will address the differences and similarities between traditional and modern-day shamans, as well as the proliferation of so-called "plastic shamans" and the dangers they signify.

Training of the Shaman

Call to the Path

The vocation of the shaman is not taken up lightly. It is not something that can be learned in a weekend retreat or by reading books. The vocation needs years of intense, narrow-minded focus and diligent study. And one is usually only called to the path after some kind of harrowing ordeal. The process of being called to the path of the shaman generally involves some kind of dramatic event; there isn't room here to categorize all of these experiences, though the below paragraphs will outline a few of the most exemplary.

The most simple and straightforward way to be led to the path of the ayahuasquero (ayahuasca shaman) is to be called by the plants themselves. Someone may suffer some kind of injury that may require them to drink the medicine as a part of their healing journey. Over the course of their visionary experience, the spirits of the sacrament may come forward and instruct the patient. When the spirit of the ayahuasca informs someone that it is their duty to take up the path of the ayahuasquero, it is considered terrible luck to refuse.

Someone may also be chosen for this sacred occupation through the course of an initiatory illness. This illness usually brings someone to the verge of death and shows them visions of the spirit world. When the person returns to waking consciousness, their training begins.

Close brushes with death are a common sign of the calling of the shaman. Illness is one means of initiation. Among some of the peoples of the upper Amazon, those who have survived attacks by jaguars are considered to be the best candidates for the job. This is due to the jaguar spirit's close association with the medicine, and the fact that it is believed many shamans can shapeshift into the form of a jaguar.

The Years of Training

Once the student has been called to the path, they must undergo an extended period of intense training. This may involve being isolated from the rest of their community, sometimes for years at a time. One shaman, Emilio Gomez, was born in the Peruvian Amazon. He suffered an accident and had to drink ayahuasca as part of his healing process; during the experience, he was called to the medicine path by the spirit of the plants.

Emilio had to remove himself from his community for three years. This period of separation allowed him to clear his mind of all attachments to the ordinary world. Whether someone lives in New York or the Amazon jungle, there is a rhythm and a pace to everyday life. There are tasks that need to get done, things that they worry about, and material concerns to absorb them. When someone is focused on the day-to-day business of living in the everyday world, the mind is filled up. There is no mental space in which to absorb spiritual wisdom.

When someone removes themselves from everyday life for a period of time, the concerns of everyday life begin to fall away. When someone does not have to worry about working to bring home dinner, or is not hung up on their neighbors gossiping about them, mental space is freed up. By immersing oneself in silence, eventually, silence falls In the mind. Once that silence was achieved, Emilio was able to receive the wisdom of the plant kingdom.

In order to open his mind and his body up to the teachings, he had a very strict regimen that he had to undergo. The first set of restrictions he had to undergo was dietary. The diet consisted for the most part of plantains and fish. He could eat some meat, but only jungle birds. And even then, he was only allowed to eat the meat of the left breast. He was not allowed to eat any other kind of meat.

He was also banned from drinking alcohol or having sexual contact during those three years. He had no contact with fertile women. His food was delivered and prepared either my a young girl or a woman past menopause. Whatever food he did not eat was collected and then destroyed; this way, no other person or animal would eat it.

The specialized diet required and the regimen of abstinence is much like that which is required of the patient seeking ayahuasca treatment. The diet allows for a "clearing out" of the body that opens the mind up more easily to the visions of the spirits. Though similar to the regimen a patient would undergo, the regimen for shamanic training is much more intense. It is taught that sexual contact gives off a "smell" that the sacred plants do not like, and thus avoid. For someone to fully receive the teachings of the plants, they must avoid sexual contact so that this "smell" does not linger on them, and does not drive away the spirits of the plants. Both sex and alcohol are things that the many cultures believe cloud the mind and prevent one from looking beyond material reality. If someone's most pressing concern is figuring out how they are going to seduce the person they find most attractive or waiting for the weekend so that they can get drunk, their minds are not focused on spiritual concerns. Once these pollutants are removed, the water clears.

During the three-year period, Emilio would wander the jungle in order to learn the wisdom of the plant spirits. In addition to his wanderings, he drank ayahuasca every two weeks as a part of his instruction. Through the consistent ingestion of the brew, he learned the terrain of the spirit world and how to navigate it. He learned about the nature of spirits, including those beneficent spirits who seek to help the shaman on their path, and the malevolent spirits that seek to hinder them. Some of those malevolent spirits were the spirits of enemy shamans, either from other tribes or the spirit world that would try to pierce his body with a kind of magical dart. This dart would allow the enemy shaman to leech his strength, or perhaps even kill him. The beneficent spirits were sometimes helpful shamans, but the majority were plant spirit teachers.

While drinking the ayahuasca, he received instruction from the spirits. Over the course of the three years, Emilio was taught roughly sixty sacred songs or *icaros*. These sacred songs were revealed to him by the plant teachers themselves. These sacred songs are extremely important tools in the shaman's tool bag. The icaros allow the shaman to manipulate the energy of a session and to guide it, like a boat. Depending on the needs of the patient and the individual circumstances, a shaman will choose to use a specific icaro.

Initiation

Once the period of three years had ended, Emilio was freed from his isolation. He was initiated into the station of the shaman and allowed to begin practicing. He used the sacred songs he had learned to accomplish many things, such as bringing the game for hunting, boosting the power of his healing remedies, and repelling the attacks of enemy shamans.

He was allowed to begin to practice fully as a shaman within his own right. Yet that does not mean he is sent off into the community unsupervised. The young shaman is still inexperienced in helping others, despite the amount of knowledge they have gained from the plant nation. Young shamans that are freshly released from their training period are placed under the tutelage of an elder shaman. This elder shaman helps to guide them as they gain confidence and experience assisting their patients.

The shaman at this point is much like a student in medical school who has begun clinicals. They have gained a vast amount of knowledge through many hard years of diligent study. However, their ability to put that knowledge to use is still shaky, at best. This is where the supervising doctor comes in. The young student observes this expert in the field as he interacts with patients, and learns from his example. Eventually, the doctor allows the medical student to step up to the plate and begin to administer to patients firsthand. Even this, though, is still closely supervised.

Just as a hospital would not allow a student with only classroom learning to perform a surgery, so in traditional societies a student fresh from the jungle is not allowed to administer to patients unsupervised. The elder shaman not only acts as a guide and a teacher for the newly minted shaman but also steps in to prevent errors that could potentially harm the patient. This system of indigenous mentorship has allowed many kinds of practices and techniques to be passed down through the oral tradition for thousands of years, facilitating the preservation of knowledge and keeping alive a vital esoteric lineage

Traditional Protocols

Thus far, this chapter has addressed how the shaman is chosen, what their training consists of, and the system of mentorship they undergo. While alluded to, it has yet to directly address the role of the shaman in everyday life in the upper Amazon, the problems that they are frequently called to address, and the tools and techniques that they use to address those problems. These subjects and others will be addressed below.

The shaman serves a vital function to the everyday life of their communities. This is represented even in the architecture and layout of the villages in which they live. Villages in the jungle tend to be fairly compact, with all of the residents living near each other. At the center of the village is a building called a maloca. The maloca is a kind of longhouse that is used by many different tribes of indigenous people across the Amazon. The maloca occupies the center of the village and is the most important place in village life. It is at the maloca that the shaman performs the ayahuasca ceremonies and attends to their patients.

The shaman serves many roles and wears many hats. They are not only responsible for presiding over ayahuasca ceremonies and seeing to patients with spiritual ailments. They also serve as healers of a more everyday variety. During their time in the jungle, the student is not only required to master the lore of the spirits, but also the functional medicine of the plants that they are surrounded by. The shaman learns not only how to traverse the world of the spirits, but also how to use medicinal plants to heal wounds and to attend to the injured and the sick. The shaman also acts as the glue that holds the social life of the village

16

together. They may be called upon to give advice, to read the future, or to diffuse tense situations between two or more parties. All of these things are the domains of the shaman, as it is believed that on occasion enemy shamans will send dark spirits to disrupt village life and to cause chaos and disorder.

In the simplest terms, the shaman is the primary line of defense between the village and the chaos of the world. With their supernatural powers, they are able to tap into the world of the spirits and to solve a huge array of problems. If the community is compared to a living organism, then the shaman serves as the immune system, keeping the organism healthy and safe by keeping out detrimental influences and energies. In a purely material sense, life in the Amazon is harsh and often unkind. In order to have some kind of peace of mind, it would make sense that the indigenous people of the Amazon would construct a cosmology in which the chaotic events of their lives were attributed agency. And it would also make sense that their worldview and spiritual life would evolve so as to give its primary wielder (the shaman) the power to diffuse those negative agents.

Uses for Ayahuasca

Ayahuasqueros use sacred medicine to address a wide variety of concerns in the life of the village. They may use ayahuasca as a part of the diagnosis and treatment of individual patients. They may use the sacred plant to communicate with the gods to discover the source of environmental problems, such as fire or drought, and how to alleviate them. They may also use it to venture into the spirit world to do battle with enemy shamans and dark sorcerers who are attempting to do them or their village harm.

In their function as doctor, the shaman uses ayahuasca for two purposes. The first is to discover the source of the illness. The shaman sits in consultation with the patient and ingests the medicine. Then, utilizing the visionary effects of the plant, they use their enhanced vision to peer into the patient's body. The ayahuasca allows the shaman to see illness, spirits, or dense energies attached to the body of a person with regular vision they would not see anything at all.

Then, the shaman may ingest ayahuasca in order to consult with the spirits as to the most effective form of treatment for the individual. If the person has fallen ill because a portion of their soul has been taken, then the shaman must undergo a journey into the spirit world to retrieve the lost part of the patient's soul. If the person has a dark spirit attached to their body, then the shaman may consult with their helping spirits or deities to create a treatment plan for the patient.

If larger problems begin to trouble the village, such as lack of game or drought, the shaman may also ingest the ayahuasca to consult with the spirits and the gods. From these divine conversations, the shaman seeks to discover the cause of the trouble. If the cause is an earthly one, such as problematic behaviors or disputes, then they are addressed by earthly means. If they are caused by spiritual infringements, then the shaman will address them through spiritual means. One such example of this is when enemy sorcerers or shamans try to attack the shaman.

Tools and Techniques

The shaman has many tools that they use in their practice. This section will only be looking at a few that have direct correlations to the ayahuasca ceremonies. The first is the shaman's spirit helpers that assist them in their work. The second is the icaros that the plant teachers gift to them. The third is the skill of shape-shifting. The fourth and final tool that is commonly used by the shaman in relation to ayahuasca is the skill of shamanic flight.

Each shaman attains spirit helpers that act as assistants in the spirit realms. As stated in the first chapter, the four archetypal animals that act as assistants are the condor and eagle, the snake, and the jaguar. These helpers have several functions. During the ayahuasca ceremony, they can act as guardians and threshold keepers. They can offer advice and guidance to the shaman. Perhaps most importantly, they protect the shaman's spirit-body has the shaman travels the unearthly realms, to prevent enemies or malevolent spirits from doing harm.

The second tool is the icaros that the plant spirits gift the shamans with. The icaros will be covered in-depth in a later chapter, but suffice to say they are perhaps the most important skill that the shaman will learn outside of the ayahuasca recipes.

Many shamans also gain the skill of shape-shifting, which is the third skill. This skill allows the ayahuasquero to embody the traits of the animal whose form they take on. The most common forms are that of the jaguar, but also of birds. During one ayahuasca session, a patient was having a difficult time. The shaman came up to him and placed their hand on his chest. The patient reported feeling the shaman's hand turn into a jaguar paw.

The spirit helpers and the skill of shape-shifting are directly linked to the fourth skill, which is shamanic flight. Shamans are able to either take on the form of a bird or ride a bird who acts as a guide to access the spirit realms. The shaman seeks entry into these realms for a variety of reasons, such as needing to consult with deities or searching for a lost piece of someone's soul.

Marks of a True Shaman

Ayahuasca has become much more popular among people in the Western world. It is no longer an esoteric secret hidden away in the Amazonian jungles. However, with the profusion of interest has also come a profusion of people looking to exploit often gullible Westerners out of their money.

A true ayahuasquero has a few key qualities. First among them is demanding that the would-be patient undergo the preparation regimen. The preparation regimem includes a specialized *dieta* for at least a month beforehand and abstaining from alcohol and sex for a prescribed period of time. All of these elements are vital to clearing the body and opening the mind so that the medicine will work with the body. Any shaman who does not ask their students to prepare does not have their patients' best interests at heart.

Another key trait to an authentic shaman is that an honest ayahuasquero takes the time to diagnose and assess the patient. If an alleged shaman is merely handing out medicine and laying people down, they are not helping the patient's healing process. In order to know how to help the patient, the shaman first must have some kind of conversation with them. If there is a language barrier, then the shaman must somehow be made aware of their inner struggles and challenges.

There are some places that offer "day trip" excursions, and ferry unknowing tourists to "shamanic ceremonies," which really entail an assembly-line like mentality. The shaman will put on some kind of performance, hand out the medicine, lay the tourists down, and send them on their way when they are done. While this is sometimes just a case of tourists getting tricked out of their money, there is also a more nefarious dimension. It is believed that a sorcerer masquerading as a shaman can beguile tourists into taking ayahuasca and them sap their life force while they are vulnerable. For this and all of the other reasons listed above, finding an authentic practitioner to guide one's experience is probably the most important thing one could do when looking to have an ayahuasca experience.

Modern Shamans and Treatment Centers

Westerners did not encounter the sacred brew known as ayahuasca until several thousand years after it had been discovered in the first place. The first Westerners entered the Amazon in the 16th century. Of course, the first point of contact was with Christian missionaries, who characterized the brew and the ceremonies surrounding it as being "of the devil." They believed that the indigenous people were Satan-worshippers due to their respect for the anaconda and other snake spirits and that the hallucinogenic brew was part of a culture of witchcraft.

Few Westerners had ever heard of the medicine until fairly recent history, and most of those who had encountered it prior to the 20th century were of the same opinion as those early Christian missionaries. The modern fascination with the sacrament is an extremely recent occurrence.

Famous American poet Allen Ginsberg was among the first Westerners to take an interest in the plant. He trekked deep into the Peruvian rainforest and found a mestizo ayahuasquero to administer the brew. Ginsberg had terrifying visions of death, which he wrote about in *The Yage Letters*. Ginsberg was followed nine years later by brothers Dennis and Terrence McKenna, who would become two of perhaps the most famous psychonauts of all time. The two brothers were grieving the death of their mother. They had searched for answers in many of the world's spiritual traditions and had still been left with questions. Eventually, they decided to put all of their bets on the truths revealed in the psychedelic experience.

They trekked for four days into the jungle, and eventually crossed the Columbian border. The two bearded brothers looked like quite the stereotypical hippies and had collected an assembly of cats, dogs, and monkeys on the trek through the jungle. This parade arrived at the village of La Chorrera and was met with a mixture of cautiousness and amusement. If they were looking for a psychedelic experience, they had found one. *Psilocybin cubensis*, a hallucinogenic species, grew on piles of cattle dung in the fields; hammocks lined the field, set up for people to lie in while tripping.

The first Western academic to study the medicine was Richard Evans Shultes of Harvard. Shultes was the founder of the field of ethnobotany and spent much effort researching and writing about the plant. One of Schultes's students brought a cutting of the ayahuasca vine back to the University of Hawaii in 1976. This was coincidentally the same time and place that Dennis McKenna was studying to get his MA.

The writings of these psychonauts and academics helped to draw international attention to this South American jungle plant. The so-called "ayahuasca boom" began in the 1990s. Westerners, starved of the sacred, began to flock to the jungle seeking the healing that their spirit-starved culture could not offer them. In the early days of the ayahuasca boom, those early seekers had to trek into the jungle and drink the medicine in a traditional maloca under a thatched roof. In the year 2000, though, something began to change. Ayahuasca retreat centers began to crop up. The early 2000s saw a boom of ayahuasca centers being founded, centered in the city of Iquitos in Peru. At the turn of the millennium, there were no treatment centers. Now, there are more than one can count. There is a huge range of variety in these centers. Some are simple affairs where a patient rents a hut in the jungle and then gathers at the maloca every other day for a ceremony. Some centers are huge, sprawling complexes have more in common with spas than they do with the traditional lineage of the ayahuasca plant.

These centers are usually, though not always, run by white non-Natives. These centers employ indigenous ayahuasqueros to administer to their Western patients. It is useless to try and count how many hundreds have sprouted in the Amazon. For a point of reference, there are dozens of listicles on wellness and healthy living websites ranking the best ayahuasca retreat centers along with matcha powders and yoga mats. Retreat centers charge anywhere from several hundred to several thousand dollars for the experience, with time frames ranging from a few days to several months. The most intense of these regimens will have the patient ingesting ayahuasca every other night; however, the exact details of the frequency and protocol vary from center to center.

While the commodification of ayahuasca is an ongoing debate in the upper Amazon, the healing that people find in the jungle is real. However, there are charlatans who seek to pretty on Westerners entering the jungle. These tourists, eager for an authentic connection to fill the spiritual void of Western culture, are sometimes eagerly taken in by people with less-than-noble intentions.

There are two kinds of people that occupy the category of a charlatan. The first is the plastic shaman or a Westerner who takes up the label as a shaman and administers the medicine without the intense years of training most shamans to endure. Sometimes these people are derisively called "yogahuascas." However, this kind of charlatan is more likely to be encountered in New York or San Francisco, not in the jungle proper.

The second kind of charlatan is the indigenous or mestizo person who is likewise unaccredited. His ceremonies usually involve no preparation and have more of a showmanship aspect than one of actual healing. There are tour offices in major Amazonian cities with tri-fold guidebooks advertising the best ayahuasca day-trips for wide-eyed tourists to visit. If a tourist should find their way into one of these offices, they may find themselves signing up for such an experience, oftentimes advertised as an afternoon excursion. For a fee, they will be placed on a bus with several other tourists and driven down to a residence of the "shaman," who will perhaps put on some kind of performance for them, give them a dose of ayahuasca, and send them away in a few hours once the medicine wears off.

Such false shamans do not ask their patients to prepare with specialized diet or abstinence regimens, do not take the time to get to know or diagnose their patients and do not offer any time for integration and healing once the experience has ended. At the very least, the tourist will leave without having gotten the healing that they were looking for. At worst, the false shaman will have stirred up trauma in their subconscious, without taking the proper measures to process and release it. It is a wonder that there are not more tales of a mental breakdown associated with improperly administered ayahuasca. Authentic shamans cannot be found on a trifold in a tour office advertising bus service.

It is not only false shamans that pose a danger to the unwary Western tourists in search of healing. There is also the danger of additives to the brew itself. Toé, also known as *Brugmansia suaveolens*, is one such additive. Toé is a powerful additive; even the most experienced shamans will only use in tiny amounts and only in special circumstances when they need to enhance their visions. It takes decades of working with the medicine before most practitioners feel competent enough to handle this additive. Toé is also known as angel's trumpet and is an incredibly potent member of the poisonous nightshade family.

However, false shamans will add toé to their brews, because it gives incredibly intense hallucinations. The visions of true ayahuasca may be subtle, or the experience may not have a visual component at all; a patient may have a purely physical and energetic experience of purging and processing past trauma. Ayahuasca tourists may come seeking spectacular visions, and leave disappointed if they do not get them. Therefore, toé is added to give the "Disneyland" light show effect.

Toé is incredibly powerful and dangerous. Henry Miller, a 19-year-old backpacker from Britain, died from ingesting an ayahuasca brew containing toé. It is not uncommon for patients to die from an incorrectly calculated dosage of toé. Finding an honest and qualified ayahuasquero is the single most important thing one can do to ensure they get the healing they need without putting themselves in undue danger.

CHAPTER 3
Chemical Effects On The Body And The Brain

Thus far, the chapters have covered the cultural and historical context of ayahuasca, as well as the visionary archetypes that tend to accompany the experience. The chapters have also investigated the credentials and training of shamans, as well as the dangerous and sometimes deadly consequences of being taken in by a deceptive or fraudulent shaman. It is important, now, to understand now only the context of the medicine, but the components of the brew itself. The following chapter will delve into the plant itself. The upcoming sections will provide information on the most common components of the ayahuasca brew, including but not limited to: botanical information, chemical composition, and interaction with brain chemistry. Later, there will also be a brief description of the most common additives to the brew, their reason for inclusion, and their effects.

Common Components

There exists in the upper Amazon a breathtaking array of cultural and linguistic diversity. With that incredible amount of diversity in people comes an attendant diversity in cultural practices, of which the brewing of ayahuasca is one. There is no one universal combination of plants or brewing technique. Rather, each tribe has its own unique interpretation of the core recipe. At the core of that recipe is, of course, the ayahuasca vine. This vine is usually combined with one of two plants. The first of these is chacruna; the second is chagropanga. Depending on the cultural group and local ecology, either of these two may be preferred.

Ayahuasca Vine (Caapi, Yage, Natema, etc.)

Culturally, the indigenous people of the Amazon hold that this is the most essential component of the brew. The plant's scientific name is *Banisteriopsis caapi*. It is a twining vine that twines around other plants and relies on them for support. *Banisteriopsis caapi* can grow up to almost a hundred feet long. The vine does not often produce flowers; however, when it does bloom, it tends to occur around the month of January. *Banisteriopsis caapi* takes at least five years to reach maturity and usability.

People who harvest will generally take the majority, if not all, of the vine. It is generally hacked with a machete into smaller, manageable lengths and then placed into sacks. The roots are left in the ground so that the vine can recover. As ayahuasca has grown in popularity, harvesters have had to venture farther and farther into the jungle to find it. Each recipe varies in the exact amount of vine they require. One shaman reported that he requires about thirty kilograms of the raw vine to produce one to two liters of brew.

Though considered to be the most important component of the brew, ayahuasca does not actually contain any hallucinogenic agents. *Banisteriopsis caapi* contains beta-carbolic alkaloids. The three alkaloids are harmaline, harmine, and tetrahydroharmine. The active hallucinogenic component is taken from other plants; that component is dimethyltryptamine (DMT).

Normally, the body releases an enzyme called Monoamine oxidase that breaks down DMT before it can affect the brain. The beta-carbolic alkaloids act as Monoamine oxidase inhibitors (MAOIs). By inhibiting the body from releasing the enzyme that breaks down the hallucinogenic component, the ayahuasca vine enables the body to metabolize it so that the DMT can cross the blood-brain barrier.

Though *Banisteriopsis caapi* has not been demonstrated to have hallucinogenic effects when ingested in isolation, there is believed to be some net effect. Many animals, such as jaguars, have been observed chewing on *Banisteriopsis caapi*. Animals on other continents have also been observed chewing on and ingesting plants that contain MAOIs. The resultant observable effects are lessened motor control, erratic movements such as walking backwards or sudden jumping, swaying, and muscle tremors. It is hypothesized that the source of these effects is an increased sensitivity to serotonin brought on by the MAOI.

Chacruna

The second most common addition to the ayahuasca brew is a plant known colloquially as "chacruna." This colloquial name is derived from the Quechua verb "chaqruy," which means "to mix," as this plant is mixed in with *Banisteriopsis caapi* to create the ayahuasca brew. The scientific name for this plant is *Psychotria viridis*.

Psychotria viridis is a small perennial shrub in the family *Rubiaceae* and is related to the coffee plant. It produces both flowers and cherries in a manner that is similar to its relatives in the *Rubiaceae* family. This plant is a small tree that is perhaps more accurately described as a large shrub; it grows no larger than fifteen feet tall. Chacruna is easily cultivated by taking cuttings of wild shrubs and allowing them to root in the soil.

The leaves are slender and turn a dark reddish-brown color when dried. The leaves are the component that is harvested for use in the ayahuasca brew. Collection methods vary, but it is typically a ceremonial affair. One shaman reported that there are ceremonial songs that must be sung to the plant while harvesting and that one should only remove leaves from the lowest branches of the shrub. Tobacco smoke may be blown on the plant as a kind of payment. The leaves in isolation are used by the indigenous people to purify the intestines and to cure migraine headaches. It is likely through experimentation that the potent mixture of *Banisteriopsis caapi* and *Psychotria viridis* was discovered.

The leaves of the chacruna plant contain DMT. When combined with the MAOIs present in *Banisteriopsis caapi*, the breakdown is slowed enough so that the DMT can cross the blood-brain barrier. This chemical gains access to the brain easily due to the fact that it is structurally analogous to serotonin and melatonin. It then interacts with and stimulates the brain's serotonin (5-HT) receptors, which is where the effects begin. DMT taken in isolation intravenously or via inhalation is one of the most powerful psychedelics in the world, though the effects are extremely short-lived—generally a half an hour or less. When combined with the MAOIs in ayahuasca, the experience can last anywhere from six to twelve hours. The concentration of DMT per milliliter varies anywhere from .16mg per milliliter and 14.15mg per milliliter of brew.

Chagropanga

Banisteriopsis caapi is considered an essential element of the brew and provides the beta-carboline alkaloids; the other key part of the brew, the DMT-containing element, can be derived from multiple different plants. The two most common DMT-containing plants are chacruna, or its counterpart, chagropanga. Chagropanga's scientific name is *Diplopterys cabrerana*. Though some localities may use a third DMT-bearing plant not listed here as a source for the brew, chacruna and chagropanga are by far used most often.

Though a distinct plant, in some parts of Ecuador chagropanga, is also known as chacruna; the terms are used interchangeably by some groups to mean any DMT-bearing plant mixed in with the ayahuasca vine. Whereas chacruna is a small shrub, chagropanga is a woody, crawling vine. The vine is easily propagated, and cuttings can be taken and either rooted directly into the soil or placed in water.

The chemical composition of chagropanga is slightly more complex than its sister plant chacruna. The leaves of chacruna contain a simple version of the DMT molecule. The chemistry of chagropanga contains not only N, N-DMT and 5-MeO-DMT, but also N-methyl tetrahydro-beta-carboline. Whereas chacruna entirely requires the beta-carbolines lent from the ayahuasca vine, chagropanga has some of these chemicals already present in their molecular structure.

The N-methyl tetrahydro-beta-carboline prevents the body from destroying the DMT and allows it to cross the blood-brain barrier. When combined with the beta-carbolines in the ayahuasca vine, this amounts to a higher number of MAOIs than brews containing the only chacruna. Because brews containing chagropanga have a higher number of MAOIs, DMT is not only active for longer in the body, but its effects are also more powerful.

Not only is there a higher number of MAOIs in brews containing chagropanga, but the plant also contains 5-MeO-DMT. This form of DMT is not known for its visionary effects. Rather, it causes changes in sensation, emotion, and conception.

In terms of how this difference plays out in the experience of the brew, patients have reported that chagropanga gives a slightly darker (though not sinister) and more complex visionary experience than chacruna. For beginners who are new to the experience, shamans will generally recommend the less-demanding journey provided by a brew only containing chacruna. Brews that contain chagropanga tend to be more potent, powerful, and demanding on the patient's psyche.

Other Additives

The core of any brew will almost always be the ayahuasca vine and either chacruna or chagropanga. However, some shamans add other elements to their brews to achieve specific effects when required. There are many plants that may be added into the brew, but the following section will cover only three. The first is known in the Amazon as *floripondia*. The second is a plant well-known to the Western world, tobacco. The third and final common additive is known as *chiric sanango*.

The first, known as floripondia or toé, has the scientific name *Brugmansia suaveolens*. It is known colloquially in the Western world as Angel's Trumpet. It is an extremely powerful and dangerous additive to the ayahuasca brew. By no means should it ever be taken by a novice patient. Though its visionary effects are spectacular, every part of this plant is poisonous. Whenever a report appears on the news of a tourist dying after drinking ayahuasca, it is almost invariably due to drinking a brew that was tainted with toé. Other side effects of toé can include muscle paralysis and tachycardia.

Another common additive to the ayahuasca brew is *Nicotiana rustica*, commonly known as tobacco. It is known colloquially in the Amazon as mapacho. This plant is known for its slight mood elevation effects, to which smokers can attest. It has no standalone psychedelic components. It does contain MAOIs and can increase the potency of the brew. The shamans also use mapacho as a spiritual cleansing agent during the ceremony and may purify the space as well as the body, wherein it acts as a purgative. Mapacho can also increase awareness and attention, making the patient more sensitive to the brew's effects.

The final plant commonly added to the mixture is known as *chiric sanango*. This plant's scientific name is *Brunfelsia grandiflora*; it is a small flowering shrub that is a member of the nightshade family. It is considered an incredibly powerful spirit and is considered a master plant spirit. Some patients are prescribed a diet largely consisting of this plant for an entire month to help heal specific physical and emotional traumas.

Chiric sanango contains the same tropane alkaloids as toé but is far less toxic and dangerous. The shamans will add it in order to allow the brew to be blessed by the animal and plant spirits.

Physical Effects

The first part of this chapter covered the most common components of the brew, as well as their physical characteristics, chemical structures, and reasons for inclusion into the brew. The following section will detail the effects that brew has on the physical body. These most notable physical effects that a patient may note after taking ayahuasca are: purging, changes to heart rate and blood pressure, rises in sensory acuity, and dizziness and disorientation. While this chapter focuses on the physical effects, a detailed exploration of the psychological aspects of the experience will be provided in a later chapter.

Purging

Perhaps the most notorious physical aspect of the ayahuasca experience is the infamous purge. People typically purge through the mouth in the form of vomit; however, some people may also experience purging in the form of diarrhea. There is an immensely important spiritual and psychological aspect to the purge that will be covered in a later chapter. This section will detail the physical aspects of the purge and the mechanism that causes it.

The area of the brain (or more accurately, brainstem) that controls the urge to vomit is called the postrema. Ayahuasca aggravates the 5HT3 serotonin receptors in the postrema; these same receptors also exist in the gut. Aside from interacting with these receptor sites in the gut and brain, it also increases serotonin levels in both of these areas. Because the interactions with these receptor sites are so intense, the vomiting that patients experience on ayahuasca is usually far more powerful and violent than typical vomiting. Due to the way that ayahuasca also stimulates the gut, it can cause diarrhea in addition to vomiting.

When ayahuasca has been taken in freeze-dried form, less purging has been noted. Thus, it could possibly be extrapolated that something about taking the medicine in liquid form increases the associated purgative properties. However, while this is an interesting observation, a patient would be hard-pressed to find freeze-dried ayahuasca served in a traditional ceremonial context by a reputable shaman in the Amazon.

Aside from the spiritual dimensions of purging (to be covered later), there exists another reason for the patient to be stimulated into vomiting. The patient will drink as much ayahuasca as they can stand in terms of flavor. However, sometimes the amount that is drunk is too much for the body to handle. Once it reaches its threshold of how much medicine it will tolerate, the body will reject the remainder of the medicine by vomiting.

The noxious flavor of the brew certainly does not do anything to decrease the level of nausea. It has notes of fetid licorice and a thick syrupy texture that some liken to cough syrup.

Heart and Blood Pressure

Another common side effect of ingesting the ayahuasca brew are changes in the vascular system while under the influence of the medicine. These effects fall into two categories. First, even though patients are lying down and inactive, they may experience changes in heart rate such as speeding up and slowing down. Secondly, patients may experience increases in blood pressure over the course of the experience.

It can be extremely alarming to be lying still and to suddenly feel one's heart rate speed up. This may manifest as a slight fluttering, or as a powerful pounding in the chest. Though it may cause fear in the mind of the patient, they should prepare for this possible side effect and do their best to remain calm if this side effect should arise.

At this time there are not any clear indicators of a chemical component in the ayahuasca brew that speeds the heart rate. It is likely that the causes for raised heart rate are emotional rather than chemical. People who have heart arrhythmias should not be concerned, as ayahuasca does not chemically affect heart rate.

There is, though, a clear link between the MAOIs in the ayahuasca vine and higher blood pressure in patients. For people who have heart conditions, it is very important to adhere strictly to the preparatory diet (detailed in the following chapter) in order to avoid blood pressure complications. When blood pressure spikes mid-ceremony, it may result in a feeling of chest pain and tightness. It may even possibly result in a life-threatening blood-pressure spike. One will generally not experience this side effect as long as they prepare properly.

If a patient has a heart condition, it is highly recommended that they consult with a medical professional before taking ayahuasca. Not only is this due to the raises in blood pressure that may result, but in the dangerous interactions that blood pressure medications can have with the medicine. These complications are covered in the next section.

To summarize, people who suffer from heart conditions should consult with medical professionals before taking the medicine, as ayahuasca can cause blood pressure spikes. These potential spikes can be avoided by adhering to the preparatory diet. Those who heart arrhythmia are not at risk, as the cause for increased heart rate is not a chemical one, but rather an emotional one.

Increased Sensory Acuity

Another common physical effect of ingestion of the sacred medicine ayahuasca is an increase in sensory acuity. This includes all five of the senses: touch, taste, smell, hearing, and sight. Patients report being able to detect things that their normal senses would never be able to detect. This includes the ability to smell the faintest of odors in the jungle, feel the vibrations of ants walking on the wood of the maloca, and to see in the dark.

Many patients have the disconcerting experience of being able to see in the dark. Traditionally, this effect has been linked with the jaguar spirit and its powerful night-vision. In a purely chemical sense, this effect can be linked to the pupil dilation commonly associated with psychedelics. Pupil dilation is scientifically termed as mydriasis. Mydriasis occurs when either the iris sphincter or the iris dilator is activated by the sympathetic or parasympathetic nervous system.

These systems, controlled by serotonin, are affected by the increased serotonin levels DMT causes by agonizing the 5-HT2A receptors. Once the pupils are dilated, the eye is able to capture more light. Being able to capture more available light than normal allows the patient to temporarily experience superior night vision and lends them the ability to see in the dark.

Patients may find other senses temporarily heightened as well. This is likely due to the increased amounts of neural activity that is brought on by the medicine. Increased neural activity means that the brain has increased power to analyze and recognize input. The increase in sensory power does not mean that the patient's nose or ears have suddenly grown more powerful or acute. Rather, it means that the brain is devoted to a higher amount of resources than usual to analyzing the typical levels of input.

Our brains only have so much computing power that they can dedicate to discrete tasks. At any given moment on an average day, the nerves are providing sensory input to the brain. To avoid distractions, the brain filters out certain sensory input. For instance, one's body is constantly receiving input about the sensations of the clothing that they are wearing, but the brain filters it out to avoid distraction. The effects of ayahuasca turn off the filtering part of the brain, allowing one to fully experience the full range of the input from their five senses.

Disorientation

Another of the most common effects that patients will experience during the ayahuasca ceremony is a loss of ability to move around freely. There are three factors that contribute to this loss of mobility. Firstly, patients tend to experience changes in vision and depth perception, affecting the ability to judge space and distance. Secondly, fine motor control skills are compromised partly due to neurochemistry and partly due to muscle tremors caused by the medicine. Thirdly, ayahuasca can cause a general sense of dizziness and disorientation that can make it difficult to walk.

Ayahuasca has significant effects on the eye. It causes dilation of the pupil, giving the patient the ability to see better in the dark. However, despite the increased ability to gather light and gain visual sensory data, the brain's ability to interpret that sensory data can be skewed by the neuropharmacology of the plant. Ayahuasca can affect depth perception, making it difficult for the patient to judge distances and space. This is one reason walking and motor functions are reduced.

Ayahuasca also affects the fine and gross motor skills. Patients may experience a reduced ability to grasp items, such as a bucket or a handrail. It also affects the coordination and can make walking difficult. Most ayahuasca ceremonies encourage patients not to move during the experience. If for some reason they must, then a guide is on hand to help the patient. The brew may also cause a generalized feeling of disorientation, which stems from the copious amounts of serotonin flooding the brain. Among the problems with fine and gross motor control and changes in depth perception, part of the medicine's hallucinogenic effects can cause not only spatial and visual distortions but also changes in the brain's ability to process and categorize input, or even to locate itself in time and space.

Taking ayahuasca is a decision that one should not make lightly. Aside from the well-known hallucinogenic effects, there is a huge host of physical effects of which the novice may be unaware. These effects include changes in the brain's ability to process sensory input, leading to loss of motor control; increased heart rate and potentially dangerous changes in blood pressure, increased sensory acuity; and intense and often violent purging through both diarrhea and vomiting. All persons should consider these effects before deciding to drink the brew, and consult with a medical professional if necessary.

Chemical Interactions

The previous sections have laid out the biochemistry of the active components of ayahuasca and the way they interact with the brain. They have also discussed the common physical effects of ayahuasca. Both of these sections have laid the groundwork necessary to understand how certain medications interact with ayahuasca. Under no circumstances should anyone ingest ayahuasca while also taking any of the drugs mentioned below, as life-threatening complications may result. The below section will describe the medications and the details of the dangerous chemical interactions.

Antihypertensives and Vasodilators

These categories of drugs affect the vascular system and the pressure of the blood flowing through that system. The first of these is antihypertensive drugs or drugs that are used to control high blood pressure. These drugs may include diuretics or beta-blockers. Antihypertensives, when mixed with ayahuasca, can cause a hypotensive crisis. Blood pressure can drop to dangerously low levels, and may even be fatal.

Even without the complication of medication, ayahuasca can cause drastic blood pressure spikes. Adding any of these drugs into the mix is very dangerous. Anyone who has hypertension or hypotension should consult with a doctor before deciding to ingest ayahuasca.

The second category of drugs that affects the vascular system is called vasodilators. Just as the name suggests, these drugs dilate the blood vessels to lower blood pressure. This category of drugs does not have a direct chemical interaction with any of the components with ayahuasca. This category of the drug increases the likelihood of fainting during the experience.

While on its face this is may not seem dangerous, being unconscious after ingesting ayahuasca can be dangerous. It increases the likelihood of choking on one's own vomit, which aside from being potentially deadly, is extremely unpleasant most people would rather avoid.

Antihistamines

Antihistamines tend to be over-the-counter drugs, and they usually clear out of the system fairly quickly. Most have evacuated the system within twenty-four hours. However, to be safe, it is recommended that none of this kind of drug be taken within forty-eight hours. As long as the patient has not taken any antihistamines at least two days before ingestion, they will not suffer from the effects outlined below.

Antihistamines are dangerous in combination with ayahuasca due to the fact that they contain pseudoephedrine. This chemical can pose dangers when combined with an MAOI. The interaction between the two chemicals can cause a hypertensive crisis, also known as a spike in blood pressure. This sudden spike in blood pressure drastically increases the likelihood of suffering a brain hemorrhage or stroke. Thought not every antihistamine contains pseudoephedrine, as a rule, this class of drugs is best avoided prior to ayahuasca ingestion.

Barbiturates

Barbiturates are a class of drug that is derived from barbituric acid. These drugs act by suppressing the central nervous system to achieve a sedative effect and cause muscle relaxation. This class of drugs affects gamma-aminobutyric acid, which is a neurotransmitter that facilitates communication between nerves. Barbiturates may be prescribed to people who suffer from insomnia, headaches, or seizures.

This class of drug can increase the sedative effects of ayahuasca when the two are combined. This can be dangerous because the sedative effects do not only cause the muscles to relax. It can also cause the muscles that control breathing and the heart to cease working, leading to asphyxiation or cardiac arrest. If the sedative effect is intense enough, it can cause the patient to lapse into a coma. This class of drugs is should in no way ever be combined with ayahuasca.

The length of time that it takes for barbiturates to clear out of the system varies. Not only does it depend on the patient's height, body mass, and duration of use, but it also depends on the kind of barbiturate used. Some evacuate the body in as little as a week. Some, though, take up to six weeks to clear completely out of the system. Individual patients should consult with their healthcare provider to determine the exact length of time that detoxing will take.

SSRIs

This acronym stands for Selective Serotonin Reuptake Inhibitor. This class of drug works by preventing the neuron from reabsorbing the serotonin that is sitting between the synapses. By preventing the serotonin from being reabsorbed, the drug makes more serotonin available for use in the brain. It is named "selective" serotonin reuptake inhibitor because it only targets serotonin and no other neurotransmitters. Under no circumstances should a patient take SSRIs and ayahuasca concurrently.

This class of drug is commonly used to treat depression. Some common SSRIs include Zoloft, Prozac, and Lexapro. By allowing there to be more serotonin available for use in the brain, this class of drug can help to improve and stabilize mood. SSRIs may also be prescribed to treat other conditions, such as anxiety disorders.

Simply put, selective serotonin reuptake inhibitors prevent the brain from reabsorbing serotonin. DMT works in part by flooding the brain with serotonin. When these drugs meet in the body, it can cause an oversaturation of serotonin in the brain. This oversaturation can lead to serotonin syndrome. This syndrome can cause heightened body temperature, tremors, and sweating. It may also cause seizures, muscle breakdown, and death.

SSRIs are a class of drug that takes a significant amount of time to detox from. Most retreat centers in the Amazon require that all potential patients detox from SSRIs for at least six weeks prior to ingestion of ayahuasca. However, because this class of drugs is usually prescribed to treat depression, it is vital to consult with healthcare and mental health professionals prior to going off of them. The benefits of the ayahuasca experience should be weighed against the potential detriments to going off of the medication.

MAOIs

This acronym stands for Monoamine oxidase inhibitors. This class of drugs works by preventing the body from releasing the enzyme monoamine oxidase. Monoamine oxidase is responsible for clearing neurotransmitters out from between the neurons. These neurotransmitters include serotonin, norepinephrine, and dopamine. Because these neurotransmitters aren't destroyed by the enzyme, they are able to remain between the neuron, making more of the neurotransmitters available for use by the brain.

MAOIs work in a fashion similar to SSRIs, but instead of only targeting serotonin, they target the entire spectrum of neurotransmitters. Like SSRIs, this class of drugs is also prescribed to treat depression. Some commonly prescribed medications that contain MAOI are Marplan and Nardil.

As mentioned in the section on the biochemistry of ayahuasca, the brew works because it contains a powerful MAOI. Monoamine oxidase is the enzyme that clears out not only neurotransmitters but also DMT. The novice might mistakenly think that taking an MAOI-bearing medication would actually be beneficial, as it would prevent the body from breaking down the DMT in the brew. In truth, the result is disastrous. Because the patient already has MAOI in their system, when combined with the MAOI in the brew, it could over-saturate the brain with serotonin, leading to serotonin syndrome. The dangers of serotonin syndrome are outlined in the subsection prior to this one.

SNRIs

This acronym stands for Serotonin and Norepinephrine Reuptake Inhibitors. This class of drug works by preventing the brain from cleaning out neurotransmitters between neurons. The two neurotransmitters that SNRIs target are serotonin and norepinephrine. Allowing these two neurotransmitters to remain between the synapses has been shown to alleviate symptoms of many different kinds of conditions.

This category of drugs is not only used to treat depression and anxiety, but also conditions involving chronic pain and nerve pain. SNRIs are especially useful for people who experience chronic pain in addition to depression. Commonly prescribed SNRIs include Cymbalta and Effexor. SNRIs can cause serotonin syndrome when taken in conjunction with ayahuasca, and should not be combined under any circumstances. SNRIs can have extremely intense withdrawal symptoms, so the benefits of the ayahuasca experience should be weighed against the difficulty of the withdrawal. SNRIs take up to two months to clear from the system.

CNS Depressants

This acronym stands for Central Nervous System Depressant. This is a class of drug that works by affecting gamma-aminobutyric acid (GABA) in the brain. CNS depressants increase levels of this chemical. GABA inhibits activity in the brain. By inhibiting brain activity, it causes a drowsy or calming effect. This class of drugs contains sedatives, hypnotics, and tranquilizers.

CNS depressants are used to treat anxiety disorders, panic, sleep disorders, and acute stress reactions. CNS depressants are a broader category that contains several of the contraindicated drugs listed previously, such as barbiturates. The first category of CNS depressants is benzodiazepines, such as Valium, Klonopin, and Xanax, which are used to regulate mood. The second category of CNS depressants is non-benzodiazepines sedative hypnotics, such as Ambien and Lunesta, which are used to help treat insomnia.

These medications achieve their effects by causing muscle relaxation and slowing bodily functions such as breathing and heart rate. As previously stated in the section on barbiturates, it is extremely dangerous to combine these drugs with ayahuasca due to the fact that ayahuasca amplifies the depressant effect. It can cause dangerous slowing of the heart rate and breathing—and may even cause those functions to stop altogether. This is a potentially deadly side effect.

It takes between three and four weeks to detox off of CNS depressants. Some CNS depressants take longer to clear from the body than others. It would be beneficial to speak to one's healthcare provider to determine the exact length of the detox associated with their specific medication.

The chemical structure of the medicine ayahuasca is complex, with an intricate web of effects on the body, brain, and psychology. Due to the complexity of this medicine, it is incredibly important to understand the chemical processes that affect the biochemical mechanisms that underlie the experience. Not only is it important to understand how the medicine affects the brain, but it is also vital to understand how the chemical mechanisms of the medicine interact with prescription drugs.

If a potential ayahuasca patient is taking any kind of prescription medication, it is extremely important to check to ensure that their medication is not contraindicated with ayahuasca. If it is, then the patient must determine if drinking ayahuasca is worth the physical and mental efforts of detoxing from the drug. If they determine that it is, then they must allow adequate time for the medication to clear from their system before drinking the sacrament.

CHAPTER 4
Preparation

The previous section outlined the complex chemical interactions that can occur when one ingests ayahuasca. Preparation is not only a matter of showing one's seriousness about the medicine but is also often medically necessary to prevent dangerous side effects. The preparation regimen for ayahuasca is one of the most intense such regimens of any sacrament. With other psychedelics such as psilocybin or LSD, virtually no preparation is necessary before one dives into the experience. With this sacrament, though, there are many steps and protocols that must be followed in order to engage properly with the experience. Among those protocols are prescriptions for diet and behavior that must be adhered to, including restrictions on certain kinds of food, refraining from sexual activity, and abstaining from medications, alcohol, and other kinds of intoxicants.

Intentions and Expectations

Before someone can begin preparing, they have to first be fully aware of what they're getting themselves into. Most people who decide to drink ayahuasca do so because they have some kind of preformed notion about what the experience will be like. These people may be of a few different varieties. They may be looking for some kind of exotic "trip," and come to the jungle purely for a psychedelic experience. They may just be curious as to what the experience is like. They may be aware of some deep-rooted need for healing in their psyche.

Unrealistic Expectations

When someone decides to go down to the Amazon in order to drink ayahuasca, normally they have some kind of preconceived notion as to what the experience will entail. These notions can not only end up preventing someone from fully immersing in the experience as it is but actually, contribute to a larger pattern of danger by unprincipled ayahuasqueros.

If someone flies to a different country and spends several thousand dollars on a retreat, often they have certain expectations. These expectations usually entail some variety of grand vision or direct experience with the nature of reality or the godhead. If someone who spends a month of their time and thousands of dollars does not get this experience, they may feel that both their time and money were wasted.

This idea is dangerous for many reasons. First and foremost, it contributes to the problem of unscrupulous ayahuasqueros adding *Brugmansia suaveolens,* or toé, to their brew. Toé is capable of bringing on fantastic visions. It is also extremely dangerous and not uncommonly causes life-threatening side effects and death. False shamans who want to "give people their money's worth," and possibly create return customers, will value the increased revenue flow over their patients' safety and well-being. Until there is a widespread understanding of the sometimes underwhelming nature of the visions for the novice users, there will be a demand for a spiked brew.

What Ayahuasca is, and What it Isn't

There are many things that ayahuasca is. And there many things that ayahuasca is not. First and foremost, working with the medicine of ayahuasca is not simple, nor is it easy. The visions are rarely straightforward, and one can be submerged in long-repressed traumas they had long thought forgotten. Being forced to relive the worst moments buried in your psyche is the least of what ayahuasca can do.

The medicine is also, sometimes, not particularly psychedelic. This may come as a crushing disappointment to those who visit the Amazon seeking grand visions. They may have an experience that is extremely emotional, purgative, or energetic, but without dazzling visuals.

Considering all of the trauma, repressed memories, and problematic patterns of behavior that ayahuasca can bring up and call out, going to the jungle is not a vacation. It is an opportunity to do exhausting, difficult, and humbling inner work. A visit to the jungle is not a relaxing experience; it is a challenging, humbling one.

Finally, ayahuasca is not always straightforward. The emotions, feelings, and insights that it brings up may seem muddled and confusing. If one is hoping for easy answers right out of the gate, this is the wrong place to look. Understanding can unfold slowly after the experience, perhaps weeks or months afterward. It requires time and patience.

Though the medicine is none of the above things, it is still extremely worth doing. For someone willing to do the work, it can provide an invaluable experience on par with years of therapy. Everyone has traumas that they have been forced to repress, due to Western society not giving them the space, tools or time they need to process properly. Ayahuasca gives the patient the ability to walk through the shadows of their subconscious and begin to clean house.

One is given the opportunity to face problematic patterns of behavior, and to understand the traumas and misguided beliefs that those harmful patterns are rooted in. Ayahuasca can also show someone where the damaged relationships in their life are that need repair, and the source of that relationship's wound. By forcing the patient to examine the repressed aspects of their subconscious and to process forgotten traumas, the medicine can facilitate great healing of the mind and give invaluable knowledge of self. Of course, the work is not done overnight, all problems solved. Rather, it gives the patient the tools to consciously work to improve themselves in their day to day lives.

Setting Intentions

Ayahuasca should not be considered as a fun excursion someone takes when they are on vacation. It is something that should be entered into with intentionality and forethought. Potential patients who enter into a ceremony just "see what it's like" may end up getting far more than they bargained for, and find themselves unable to handle what they are shown.

The spirit of the medicine can dig deep into the sludge of the unconscious mind, to help someone clear out buried traumas and unhealed wounds. Someone might find themselves reliving a terrible accident or childhood abuse. They may re-experience the parental neglect they felt as a child, with all of the overwhelming emotions they felt in the moment. These can swamp the unprepared voyager.

If one enters into the medicine without a clear intention for self-examination and healing, there is the danger of their consciousness wandering during the experience. If one's mind isn't open to the potential of healing, they conscious mind may seek to move and guide the experience and visions. This need for control may prevent the plant from being able to have an active conversation with the patient, and may prevent their healing. This is extremely disrespectful to the spirit of the medicine.

The question, then, is how does one set intentions? The art of setting intentions comes with a few thorny challenges. First and foremost, a potential patient needs to realize that if they think they are going to walk into the experience and be able to drive and control it, they are mistaken. The potential patient is better served by doing three things: intending to face their shadows, intending to surrender, and intending to be humble. It is vital that before someone enters into this experience that they acknowledge that they may be asked to face their shadow selves. These are the aspects of the self that they cringe away from, because they are unsavory, and the person wishes this part were not there at all. Deliberately deciding to be open and compassionate to this part of the self, should it arise, is the first vital intention.

The second vital intention is to deliberately decide to surrender to the wisdom of the medicine. Ayahuasca only shows what needs to be healed; whatever difficulty to arise, it must not be fought or resisted—it must simply be experienced. The final vital intention is to be humble about what is revealed. Accept whatever gift of wisdom that the plant medicine reveals, and dedicated to working with it until the wound is healed.

The Regimen

The previous section prior to this one addressed the importance of setting intentions and having realistic expectations. Deliberate forethought is a vital component of a successful ayahuasca experience. In that same vein, deliberate action and planning are also hugely important to the success of one's experience. Understanding and integrating the insights that the medicine reveals is a difficult task and requires a lot of work. However, the work doesn't just begin when one steps into the ceremony. The work begins weeks, sometimes months, beforehand. There specialized regimen that needs to be followed includes abstaining from sexual activity, certain foods, and most medications. Devoting oneself to the task of preparing shows one's seriousness regarding the healing they hope to achieve. Adequate preparation leads to a deeper experience.

Foods

The chapter prior to this detailed the chemical processes of the medicine, and the interactions that those chemical processes can have with specific medications.

This section will also look at the biochemical processes involved with ayahuasca, though this time with a focus on various kinds of foods. This section will explain what tyramine is, which foods contain it, and how this chemical interferes and interacts with the ayahuasca experience. The following section will also detail other foods that must be avoided for metaphysical reasons, as explained by shamans. Finally, the below will provide information and advice about the kinds of recipes and foods one can eat while on the preparation regimen.

Tyramine: Tyramine is a chemical that is common in certain aged and fermented foods. These foods include aged cheese, beer, cured meat, and smoked fish. On its own, tyramine has been known to cause migraines in some people. This chemical is a trace amine, and it is derived from an amino acid called tyrosine. This amino acid converts to tyramine during the process of fermentation and decay. This chemical cannot cross the blood-brain barrier. It can have sympathomimetic effects on the peripheral nervous system, though those effects are completely non-psychoactive, due to the fact that it cannot cross the blood-brain barrier. Tyramine is broken down by the enzyme monoamine oxidase (MOA). MOA is breaking down this chemical in the gastrointestinal tract, preventing toxic levels from building up in the body. Tyramine toxicity causes adrenergic hyperstimulation. The word "adrenergic" refers to the adrenal glands; put simply, the adrenal glands become hazardously overstimulated.

As previously stated, ayahuasca contains an MAOI, which inhibits the action of monoamine oxidase. Without MAO to break down tyramine, it can build up to toxic levels. When this interaction occurs, it results in a hypertensive crisis, which in turn can cause a brain hemorrhage or stroke. At the very least, it could trigger debilitating migraines.

Tyramine is found in foods that have been aged, fermented, pickled, smoked, or dried. For a start, meats that are high in tyramine include red meat and pork. Aged dairy, such as yogurt and aged cheese, is also high in this chemical. Fermented foods like sauerkraut, soy sauce, and fermented tofu should also be avoided. Alcohol also falls into this category, as it is created through the process of fermenting grains. Finally, chocolate and peanuts should be avoided, as they can contain a small amount of this chemical, though it only begins to pose a danger in higher amounts. Finally, aspartame and protein powders contain high amounts of tyramine and should be cut out of one's diet.

The above foods should be avoided due to the fact that they contain high amounts of a chemical that is dangerous when consumed prior to an ayahuasca experience. The foods listed below, however, should be avoided for different reasons, as prescribed by ayahuasqueros.

The preparatory diet prescribes that patients should not consume spicy food or food that is intensely flavored. This includes foods that are high in refined sugar, high in salt, and high in spices. Patients should also avoid caffeine, oils, and dairy.

Spiced Foods: From the perspective of a shaman, food that is intensely flavored creates an effect called *cutipado*. *Cutipado* is a widely-used term in the Amazon, though it is of Shipibo origin. It roughly translates as "bewitched." It refers to negative energy which interferes with the work of the plant medicine. Spicy foods are restricted for reasons that are less spiritual and more practical. When the purge begins, if the patient has eaten spicy foods, it will burn their sinuses and throat as they vomit, and most likely their anus if they suffer a diarrheal purge.

Salt and Sugar: The restriction on salt and sugar is also due to the fact that they make purging more unpleasant than it needs to be. This is especially true when it comes to vomit, as they can affect the consistency and flavor. If one were to eat a bowl of ice cream and drink a can of soda prior to an ayahuasca experience, they would notice their vomit would take on a syrupy, condensed consistency and an overpowering, sickly-sweet flavor.

There are many reasons to avoid certain foods prior to ayahuasca. Some are purely spiritual, while others are immensely practical. Whether one is avoiding tyramine toxicity or managing the consistency of their vomit, the diet should always be followed to the letter.

Dietary Advice

It may seem that with all of the restrictions, the only options left are bland, boring, and tasteless. That assumption is correct. Medical and chemical reasons aside, part of proving one's dedication and commitment to the medicine is cutting out foods they otherwise enjoy. However, just because a number of allowed foods is restricted does not mean that the prospective patient will starve.

There are many foods that are still on the menu. The traditional, hardcore version of the diet only allows the patient to eat green bananas, yucca, fish, rice, boiled plantains, and water. Those looking for the full, immersive experience may look into this regimen. For everyone else, foods that are still on the menu include quinoa, amaranth, fruits, vegetables, small amounts of honey, nuts, and eggs.

There are many food alternatives out there that can help someone make their way through this prohibitive period. Cashew cheese and other nut-derivative products are allowed, as long as they do not contain large amounts of salt or sugar. This is an excellent time to consider adding large, filling salads to one's diet. Aside from abiding by the regimen, adding leafy greens as a dietary staple will also do wonders for one's levels of micronutrients.

The diet can have the effect of not only adequately preparing the body for the ayahuasca experience, but also providing the patient with a greater sense of wellness and vitality. Patients may find themselves feeling revitalized, refreshed, and energized during this regimen.

To summarize, the diet can be a tricky period, as it has many requirements and can seem oppressive. Despite this, it is necessary for a variety of medical, spiritual, and practical reasons. The diet helps the patient to avoid hypertensive crisis, have an experienced untainted by *cupitado*, and have a much easier time with ayahuasca's infamous purge. It is difficult but necessary.

Abstinence

While it may seem difficult to refrain from eating certain kinds of food, other prohibitions are just as, if not more, difficult to adhere to. Of the three prohibitions (certain foods, sex, and medications), this one is the one that receives perhaps the most pushback. However, just as there are good reasons for the prohibitions on certain medications and foods, so too are there concrete concerns that sit behind this one.

Firstly, there are psychological reasons that sex and masturbation are prohibited prior to drinking ayahuasca. Procreation is one of the most basic drives that humans experience, and it is perhaps the greatest driving force in the natural world. This being the case, sex takes up a huge amount of the human brain capacity. This is a capacity of time and attention that can be freed up to accomplish other tasks.

There is a reason that monks and nuns of nearly all of the world's major traditions swear an oath of celibacy. In order to fully open themselves up to the light of the divine, monastics from these religions cut themselves off from the confusion and distraction that is sexual and romantic entanglement.

When the mind is concerned with the pleasures of the flesh, it is exponentially more difficult to connect with the light of the spirit. When one is focusing their attention on achieving a sexual connection with someone else, then their attention is turned outward. In order for ayahuasca to do its work, the person in question needs to be able to turn their full attention inward and onto the self. When one's attention is focused on someone else, then they are unable to attend to their own spiritual growth.

Just as there are reasons both practical and spiritual for abstaining from certain foods, so too are there reasons of both kinds for avoiding sexual contact. While the practical are outlined above, the spiritual shall be outlined below.

Traditional ayahuasqueros provide two reasons that sexual contact is a detriment to the ayahuasca experience. The first is that sex gives off a "smell" that is offensive to the plant spirits. While the indigenous terminology of sex having a "smell" may seem disconcerting, this can perhaps be more accurately be conceived of as energy present in the body that prevents the medicine from working correctly. There is also another reason ayahuasqueros may report that sex interferes with the medicine. Some shamans believe that the ayahuasca spirit is a woman and that she gets jealous if those who ingest the medicine have recently slept with other sexual partners.

Another useful perspective could be to consider sexual contact and masturbation as an energetic release. This not only refers to climax but also to the attention and connection forged with a partner. This energetic release depletes the energetic body. When someone is about to undergo an ayahuasca experience, they will need all the energetic reserves they can muster in order to move smoothly through the experience.

Drugs

The previous two sections detailed dietary and sexual protocols that must be strictly adhered to prior to the ceremony. This section will detail medical protocols that must be observed. As stated in the chapter on chemical effects, many medications are contraindicated, as they can have deadly interactions. Alcohol is also contraindicated, and its chemistry and effects will be explained below. Additionally, street drugs can cause dangerous interactions and should be avoided as well.

To avoid too much repetition, this section will only briefly reiterate what was stated in an earlier chapter on chemical interactions with ayahuasca. For full details, please refer to that chapter. In short, the medications listed below need to be halted prior to drinking the medicine.

The first set of complications is serotonin syndrome. The medications that can cause serotonin syndrome include selective serotonin reuptake inhibitors, serotonin norepinephrine reuptake inhibitors, and monoamine oxidase inhibitors. This complication occurs because the medications prevent serotonin from being reabsorbed into the brain; when coupled with the serotonin-flooding effects of ayahuasca, toxic levels of the neurotransmitter can accumulate, leading to death.

The second category of interaction is a hypertensive crisis. Blood pressure medications, antihistamines, and vasodilators can cause blood pressure to spike dangerously high, often leading to a stroke or brain hemorrhage. Central nervous system depressants can freeze the heart and the muscles that support breathing and can cause asphyxiation and cardiac arrest.

Alcohol is another drug that should be discontinued two weeks to a month prior to the experience. This chapter has already outlined that certain foods need to be avoided due to the presence of a chemical called tyramine. Tyramine accumulates in food that has been aged and fermented. Beer and other alcoholic beverages are, of course, made by fermenting plant matter of various kinds to convert sugar into alcohol.

Tyramine interacts with the chemicals of ayahuasca to make more of the active component (DMT) available to the brain and body. Because more DMT is able to cross the blood-brain barrier, the effects increase in strength, sometimes into the realm of the unbearable. Visions can be overwhelming, purging can be violent, and heart rate can become fast and erratic.

Alcohol has another aspect that should be considered. Like sex, it is an intoxicant. It clouds the mind and shifts one's consciousness. If one is drinking alcohol, they are reducing their ability for their mind to be clear and focused. Clarity and focus are extremely important to a successful ayahuasca experience.

Finally, non-prescribed drugs need to be avoided. For example, stimulant drugs such as cocaine, amphetamines, and methamphetamine can lead to dangerous complications involving the heart. These drugs work by triggering the "fight or flight" system in the body, either by mimicking the hormones that trigger the reaction or by enhancing the body's endogenous hormones. These drugs drastically increase the likelihood of cardiac arrhythmia.

Another category of contraindicated drugs is opiates. This includes heroin, opium, and fentanyl. The body naturally produces some amounts of opiates to block pain, calm the mind, slow breathing, etc. External opiates can overwhelm the body's capabilities and give a dangerous boost to the sedative effects of ayahuasca. Because opiates boost the levels of serotonin in the brain to block pain, it can also lead to serotonin syndrome.

Psychedelic drugs, such as psilocybin, DMT, LSD, and MDMA should also be avoided prior to ayahuasca ingestion. All of these substances create hallucinogenic effects by drastically increasing serotonin syndrome in the brain. When combined with ayahuasca, the end result will likely be a deadly case of serotonin syndrome.

There are good reasons that ayahuasqueros and retreat centers demand that their potential patients go through extensive preparation prior to arriving in the Amazon. Certain foods can cause distress in the body as well as increase the likelihood of dangerous chemical interactions. This is also the same reason intoxicants, medications, and drugs should be avoided prior. And while it will not cause a chemical interaction, sex and sexual activities draw the attention, energy, and cloud the mind. Giving up all of these things temporarily will do wonders for one's ayahuasca experience

Pitfalls

This chapter has, thus far, spent much of the previous pages describing what is necessary for the preparation for an ayahuasca experience. So far, it has described restrictions that are medical, dietary, and sexual. The final section of this chapter will elaborate on the reasons for these restrictions, and describe the consequences of what happens when one does not adequately prepare. These consequences include diminished experience, psychological distress, dangerous chemical interactions, and spiritual crisis.

Lack of Seriousness

There are many things that can be revealed by a failure to prepare. A lack of seriousness is one of them. At the very least, inadequate preparation will lead to a diminished experience and little insight. Considering the cost of time off, plane tickets, and the experience itself, this would mean thousands of dollars wasted.

Aside from the standpoint of wasted resources on the part of the patient, not following the regimen indicates a level of disregard for an ancient, powerful set of traditions. It is quite frankly amazing that the shamans of the Amazon have made this sacred visionary experience available to Westerners. Abusing that chance is outright disrespectful.

It can also be a sign that perhaps someone isn't ready for the spiritual growth that they are seeking in the first place. Being taken in by the allure of a mystical Amazonian healing ceremony is well and good, but if one isn't willing to dedicate to preparation, then perhaps they are also not ready for the difficult, slogging shadow-work ayahuasca brings to the surface.

Altered Experience

Failure to prepare properly can also change the effects of the plants on one psyche and physical body. The less troublesome of the two scenarios is that the effects of the medicine are simply diminished. The visions will not be as strong, the medicine's messages may be muddled, and the patient may emerge from the experience disappointed and without clarity.

The more dangerous of the two options is that the effects of the medicine are heightened in dangerous and unpleasant ways. The purging may be painful and difficult, and the visions may be disjointed, confusing, and terrifying. This second scenario can leave the mind of the patient broken wide open, all of their raw wounds exposed, without any of the healing they were looking for.

Offending the Spirits

The ayahuasca ceremony is fundamentally about inviting helpful guiding spirits into the space and the body to aid in healing and purging. Preparation is not only about making the physical body able to receive the medicine but also about building a relationship with the spirits. If one does not put in the effort to build a relationship with the medicinal spirits beforehand, then those spirits may simply refuse to visit and aide them during the journey.

Conversely, a lack of preparation may also offend the spirits of the medicine to such a degree that they seek to punish the would-be patient. This can lead to intense, horrifying visions meant to "scare the patient straight." The spirits can send visions ripped from the patients most repressed nightmares. Or, alternatively, the spirits may choose to confront the patient directly to admonish them about the lack of seriousness with which they approached the medicine.

Interactions

From a purely chemical standpoint, inadequate preparation can be deadly for a number of reasons. It cannot be understated that the danger of death is real with the complex chemical interactions involved in ayahuasca. At the very least, one may experience terrifying health complications such as serotonin syndrome, cardiac arrhythmia, intense and violent purging, and mild paralysis. When one goes to the Amazon for an ayahuasca ceremony, they are usually looking for healing. Without preparation, they can get just the opposite.

Aside from the individual risk to the patient, there is also a larger risk to the center or shaman from whom the patient receives the medicine. The center itself may be opened up to fire from the larger public, and perhaps even lawsuits from the family of the patient. Even if this does not occur, when someone has a negative or dangerous complication with ayahuasca due to a lack of preparedness on their part, it damages the reputation of the sacrament. A personal failure to prepare can contribute to a larger, inaccurate cultural image of this healing plant as a dangerous drug.

Time for Reflection

Aside from adhering to the dietary, sexual, and medical aspects of the regimen, there is another practice that may benefit the potential patient leading up to their experience. Many people find it immensely helpful to take up some kind of daily mindfulness or meditation practice in the weeks and months leading up to the ceremony.

There are many benefits to quiet and meditation. From a purely physical standpoint, the body is able to slow its heart rate and become more oxygenated. People who meditate have lower levels of the chemicals and hormones that cause anxiety and stress. Meditation has been linked to longer life expectancy and lower rates of diseases caused by a stress-filled life.

There are also many mental benefits of taking up a meditation practice. Lowered amounts of stress hormone allow people to find themselves calmer, more level-headed, and more resilient when stressful situations arise in their life. Moreover, when they find themselves overwhelmed or anxious, they have a practical tool to bring their minds back into equilibrium. The minds and emotions of meditators are steadier and less disturbed than those of non-meditators.

As this relates to ayahuasca, creating space in one's mind allows them to experience serenity and peace. Learning just how noisy one's own mind is can be quite a surprise for many people. In the beginning, meditation is not easy, nor is it pleasant—just like ayahuasca. People awaken to the busy, stormy nature of their thoughts and feelings. Learning to sit with the busyness eventually allows that busyness to quiet.

Becoming aware of the nature of one's own mind gives them a vital degree of self-knowledge. Meditation gives one a bird's eye view of one's own mind; to a degree, ayahuasca does as well. Learning to sit through the discomfort and difficulty of meditation is a valuable skill set that will also serve one well during the ayahuasca experience.

Finding that inner space also allows one to be self-critical, and begin to identify the shadows and traumas that may come up during an ayahuasca experience. Meditation allows one to "clean house," which is the process of learning to quiet one's mind. When the mind is cluttered and busy, it is difficult to hear anything outside of one's thoughts. This includes the words and messages of the plant medicine. If someone is unable to open a channel, the message will not come through clearly.

Conversely, if someone engages in mindfulness practice to clear out their mind, then the messages of the spirits will flow through much more easily. It can be compared to tuning a radio dial precisely. Without meditation, the messages may be filled with static; but with meditation, the dial is turned to the exact right frequency.

A contemplative practice will also aid with integration. One of the biggest challenges that people suffer comes not during the ceremony, but after. Once the messages have come through, the patient may spend weeks, months, or years sitting with the lessons that unfolded during the experience. To even the most disciplined mind, this can be a great challenge. To someone with no meditation or mindfulness training at all, it is even more difficult. Making space and quiet in one's mind will allow truths to rise to the surface as the cream rises to the top of milk. Adding a mindfulness practice to one's preparation can not only help them during the ayahuasca experience but can be a great asset for the rest of their life as well.

CHAPTER 5
The Experience

Thus far, this book has detailed much information surrounding the medicine of ayahuasca. It has detailed the cultural and mythic environment from which the ceremonies grew, the role and traits of the facilitator, the chemical effects of the plant, and the preparation regimen. All of this information leads up to the experience itself, which is what this chapter will cover. First, the below sections will explore how surrender can ease the experience. Secondly, information will be provided on the supplemental tools used in the ceremony by the shaman. Finally, this chapter will outline the psychological and visionary effects of the medicine, as well as provide a few categories of the most common kinds of ayahuasca experiences.

Surrender

Ayahuasca makes large demands on both the body and mind. It demands that one relive traumatic experiences. It demands that one be willing to look at aspects of themselves that they do not like. It demands one deal with the discomfort of prolific vomiting. Fighting against these demands just makes them harder.

Learning to let go and move with the experience is one of the best pieces of advice someone can receive going into an ayahuasca ceremony. Quite frankly, these difficult things are going to happen whether someone wants them to or not. When one agrees to drink ayahuasca, they are also tacitly agreeing to the unpleasant aspects of the experience as well. Learning to accept and move through these difficulties will make an already-challenging experience that much easier. The power of ayahuasca can be thought of as a great and powerful river; the patient is one small fish trying to fight the flow. It is better to ride the current.

The question, then, becomes: how does one surrender? There are a few ways to go about it. First and foremost, one must cultivate trust. The spirit of the medicine only wants to show what someone what they need to see in order for their own personal growth and healing. In a properly-run ceremony, the spirits will seek to help the patient reveal their traumas so that they can begin to release it. Sometimes a wound has to be reopened in order for it to heal properly. Secondly, the shadows that the medicine will reveal in one's own heart are not marks of evil or condemnation. Rather, they are neglected aspects of the self crying out for compassion and love. This understanding can help someone move through the experience more easily, and to trust the medicine's visions.

However, many people have difficulty letting go. This can perhaps stem from anxieties that are rooted in the patient's subconscious. They may have experienced some traumatic event that gives them a driving need to control their surroundings and experiences. People who suffer from control issues have some of the most difficult times in ceremony. Inability to surrender indicates a fundamental distrust of the spirits of the medicine and may affect the medicine's willingness and ability to work with the patient.

If one finds themselves unable to surrender, their experience may be likened to that of a small boat caught in a storm on the ocean. They may find themselves battered by forces beyond their control, their psyche swamped by overpowering visions, and their consciousness subsumed in chaos. To continue the water metaphor, ayahuasca is a great force, like a river.

Fighting the current, at best, will leave one in exactly the same place—just as a fish swimming against the current will not move. If the patient goes with the current, they will find themselves much farther down the path of understanding. At its most basic level, it is beneficial to cultivate the attitude that the spirits of the medicine are beneficent, and only seek to help the patient along the path of growth.

The Ceremony

There is a lot more to the ceremony than just the drinking of the ayahuasca. The shaman actively steers the experience through a variety of means. They purify and sanctify the space through the use of supplemental medicines, such as tobacco smoke and Florida water. The shaman's greatest tool, however, is the icaros. Icaros are sacred songs that channel the power of the spirits and guide the experience as it unfolds.

Tobacco

The tobacco used in the ceremony is not the same variety that one buys at a gas station convenience store. The variety of tobacco smoked by Westerners is *Nicotiana tabacum*. The sacred Amazonian variety is *Nicotiana rustica*. This second variety is referred to as *mapacho* and is used as a smudge, a purgative, and a stimulant.

The first way that tobacco is used during an ayahuasca ceremony is as a cleansing agent, prior to the drinking of the medicine. The mapacho is brewed in a bowl filled with clean water. It is similar to a tobacco tea. Once the water is infused with the essence of the tobacco, it is inhaled through the nose. The patient cups their hand and takes roughly a tablespoon of water. It is snorted once through each nostril.

It is both a stimulating agent and a grounding agent. Because it has both of these qualities, the tobacco helps the patient to have the clarity and strength for the forthcoming journey. Aside from being offered at the beginning of the ceremony, it may also be offered in the middle of the ceremony. It is especially recommended that people having a difficult experience take a second dose of tobacco.

Aside from being snorted as a stimulating agent, the mapacho is also used as a cleansing and purifying agent by the shaman. Much as the indigenous people of North America use smudge to clear out dense energies and negative spirits, so the shamans of South America use tobacco.

During the course of the ceremony, the shamans may smudge the space with tobacco to ensure that only benevolent entities remain within the space. The shamans will then typically also smudge all of the participants. The typical protocol is for the shaman to blow smoke onto the chest, back, head, and hands of the patient.

Tobacco allows the patient to be cleansed and protected both from within (through snorting) and from without (through blowing smoke). Tobacco is considered one of the master plant teachers of the Amazon.

Florida Water

This water is also known as Agua de Florida. It is named for the state of Florida, where it was once believed the Fountain of Youth resided. Florida Water has alcohol as its base ingredient, with a blend of essential oils. These oils include lavender, orange, and citrus. It is referred to as the world's most popular perfume and is used across many continents. However, the recipe varies drastically from shaman to shaman; some simply dissolve camphor and tobacco in alcohol; others have more elaborate recipes.

It is popular with the shamans of the Amazon because the plant spirits love sweet smells; the smell of the Florida water appeases them. Human smells are described by the ayahuasqueros as "acidic," and are disliked by the plant spirits. Bringing sweet smells into the space will draw in the beneficent spirits to aid in the patients' healing.

Shamans use Florida water in a few ways. Many will drink in a large quaff of the liquid and then spray it forcefully out of their mouth. This results in a fine mist. The resulting mist has purifying and cleansing qualities and is said to drive negative influences and spirits out of the space.

If a patient is having a difficult time, then the shaman may choose to cleanse them with the Florida water. The water is also used to clear dense and dark influences out from the body and energetic field. The shaman will use the same method to spray water across the patient. This process purifies the body and allows the experience to flow forward unencumbered.

The ayahuasquero can use Florida water to seal the body against negative influences. The sealing aspect also works to create boundaries between the patients' energetic fields. In order to keep one person's energy from leaking out and affecting a neighbor's experience, the shaman can set a boundary of Florida water. This ensures that each person's experience is uniquely their own and that the visions of other patients will not interfere with each individual's unique healing process.

Icaros

The icaro is perhaps the most important tools that the shamans use during the ceremony, other than the ayahuasca itself, of course. These songs are whistled and sung by the ayahuasquero prior to, during, and after the ceremony. These songs not only sound nice; they directly affect the internal experiences of the patients as they navigate the medicine's terrain.

As stated in the chapter on the role of the shaman, the songs are taught to the ayahuasquero directly by the plant spirits. Each shaman's set of songs is unique, as each ayahuasquero has a unique relationship with the plant spirits. The songs typically invoke a specific plant or animal spirit, asking them for their presence and guidance. Icaros are a measure of standing; the more songs a shaman knows, the more powerful they are considered.

Icaros are a driving force; they can be considered the propeller that drives the ceremony forward. They steer the experience, driving it deeper or higher as necessary. They induce and modulate the patients' visions. In addition to this, they also have other functions.

They can evoke helpful spirits, while also protecting the ceremony from dark spirits. The songs can intensify or mitigate the visions, depending on what is needed at the moment. They can be used to discern the cause of illnesses or conditions, as well as to discover the treatment for that illness or condition. The songs can also be used to call in healing for the sickness. They can also be used to intensify the feelings of love two people feel for each other.

While no two icaros are the same, they all have similar structural patterns. They form a distinct category or genre of sound with unique properties to affect the consciousness of patients undergoing effects of the medicine. Icaros all have a fast, rhythmic, driving quality that propels the ceremony. There is not much variation in melody, and there are usually one to three repeated phrases. The repetitive nature of the songs may help evoke theta brainwaves, deepening the experience.

The discrete States of Consciousness

The effects of ayahuasca take on many forms. The hallucinations brought on by the plant can be visual, auditory, olfactory, or tactile. The ayahuasquero will usually insist that all patients spend the majority of their time with their eyes closed. Sitting with the eyes closed allows the mind to journey into the self, and to experience the messages of the plants without extraneous input.

Psychological Effects

Perhaps one of the most difficult potential effects of ayahuasca is when the plant asks the patient to relive a traumatic event in their past. This may play out in a few different ways. For some, it may feel as if they have been transported back in time to the moment of the trauma, and are re-experiencing it as their younger self. Whether that self was a small child or a college student, it does not matter.

The patient may find themselves reviewing a traumatic event in their life as if it were on a large movie screen in their brain. This saves them from the trauma of reliving the experience, but they are still asked to critically review it.

The patient may not visually relive the experience but may feel the emotions of the event and the energy of the moment coursing through their body. The trauma locked up in the physical body is rising to the surface for the conscious mind to process; this may occur either visually or physically. Either way, it is important to remember to breathe. The body will process the trauma, and then it will flow out and away.

Another common effect of ayahuasca is the experience of time distortion. The ancient people understood that time is cyclical. Under the influence of the medicine, the brain may cease to experience time as a linear construct. This manifests differently from person to person, but there are three common experiences.

First, the patient may feel time stretching out indefinitely. They may feel the infinite nature of time and the cosmos and feel their own short lifespan to be but a blip on the face of the universe. The patient may experience the present moment as having an eternal quality, and thus begin to feel a kind of link with the infinite.

They may also experience time distortion as a compression of the events of their life. A patient who is well into middle age may gain the distinct impression that their childhood was only moments ago. Alternatively, a young patient may feel the urgency of their own aging process, and feel the years ahead of them compress.

The effects of time distortion while under the influence of the medicine greatly influence the reliving of trauma. The patient may feel as if they are time-travelling through the past events of their lives, reliving various moments as they arise in their consciousness.

Visual Effects:

Aside from the psychological effects of the medicine, such as reliving trauma and time distortion, there are the infamous visual effects that may occur while under the influence of ayahuasca. Perhaps the most famous visual pattern associated with psychedelics is the fractal pattern.

The fractal is a recurring pattern that both contains itself, and is contained within a larger iteration of itself. These dancing shapes are common in all psychedelics, from psilocybin and DMT to LSD and MDMA. The exact patterns that the patient witnesses are highly variant, and there is no one set of shapes or lines that are universally experienced. Another visual experience that the patient a patient may undergo are visitations from spirits. The spirits are usually one of the spirits associated with ayahuasca medicine, such as the snake or jaguar. However, there are other spirits associated with the medicine as well, though they are less grandiose. These include the spirits of the frog and lizard. Whatever messages the spirits impart are highly personal, and no two sets of messages are the same. No matter what they say, however, it is all intended for the deep healing and highest well-being of the patient. The patient may also experience their consciousness travelling upward and outward. Some patients travel outward out of their body and into other realms. This journey can involve visiting the underworld, which is the realm of the animal spirits and the realm of the ancestors. It may also involve travelling upwards into the heavenly realms in order to converse with gods or deities. This kind of journey usually only opens to patients who have cleared out the shadows and trauma that act as "weights" on the energetic body. Only after the patient has spent considerable time processing their trauma are they usually capable of such travels.

One kind of journey involves going out; another kind of journey involves going within. The patient may feel as if they are travelling down into the recesses of their own body. Unprocessed trauma is often locked up somewhere in the body, leading to chronic disease and ailments. The process of unlocking those traumas may cause the consciousness to travel into the body, into the place where the trauma has been stored away. A patient may experience themselves travelling down into their intestines, or into the muscles of their back. Once they reach their destination, they may experience the trauma that was locked there.

Some Categories of Experience

It is impossible to tell a potential patient what their journey will be like because each person's journey is theirs and theirs alone. However, there are some general categories of experience that hold true. These experiences range from visual to tactile to energetic. The exact categories are outlined below.

Visionary:

This category of experience usually begins with fractals and geometric shapes. Once those visuals fade, after about twenty minutes or less, the consciousness will begin to experience an intense visionary experience.

The themes of these experiences vary. Some retreat centers have reported that their patients often see images of shamans from both South American and North American indigenous traditions. Plant and animal spirits also commonly make appearances to the patient. Sometimes the patient may even see images from places as far-flung as Egypt or Atlantis. While under the sway of this kind of experience, the patient may travel out of the body and into outer space. They may even journey to the edge of the Milky Way galaxy. Some people's consciousness travels even farther than this. Shamans have reported that patients may, on occasion, travel to other dimensions and realities. Some patients thoroughly enjoy this kind of experience; for others, it may be completely overwhelming.

If the patient finds themselves drifting too far away from the body, the shaman recommends focusing on the sound of the icaros. The icaros not only drive the experience and deepen the ayahuasca experience; the songs also serve as an anchor. The consciousness of the patient can latch onto the sound of the song and follow it back to their body in the maloca, much like Hansel and Gretel following the trail of breadcrumbs out of the forest.

While some people quite enjoy this kind of experience, it is also important to remember that leaving the body may not be the most beneficial thing for one's healing. The aspects of the self that need healing are usually buried within the body, in this dimension. It is best to deal with the shadows in one's own mind and physical form first before attempting to fly off into other dimensions. The most profound healing is found in this way.

Healing:

Everyone carries wounds; it is one of the hallmarks of being human. In this category of experience, the patient begins to experience the healing of the wounds they carry through several means. They may experience healing at the hands of ayahuasca or other spirits, they may feel healing by their own powers, and they may experience healing through the process of forgiveness.

If the spirit of ayahuasca identifies a wound within a patient, she may choose to address it directly. The patient may experience themselves in a conversation with the spirit of the plant. The spirit of the ayahuasca may point out exactly what in the body, mind, or energetic field is wounded, and then perform some kind of healing on the wound.

If the spirit of ayahuasca is not the one who engages in the healing, it may be another spirit instead. A plant or animal spirit may join with the patient to help them in their healing process; the frog, lizard, or jaguar may speak with the patient—or the spirit of the tobacco or another plant teacher may work with them. Additionally, the spirits of one's own ancestors or guiding spirits may come forward to help in their healing.

The patient may, alternatively, be pointed in the direction of the wound and be told to heal the wound themselves. Instead of relying on powers outside of themselves, they may find inner reserves of strength to release whatever trauma has taken up residence in their body or energetic field. This can be an intensely emotional experience, as the person recognizes the importance of their own efforts in their healing process. The patient may be asked to forgive themselves for difficult and unsavory actions they committed in their past and buried in their subconscious. The act of forgiving the self can be a radical and powerful catalyst for personal healing.

Energetic:

This category of experience is notable for what it doesn't have, rather than what it does. People who undergo a solely energetic experience will not experience the intense visuals that most people associate with psychedelics in general, and ayahuasca in particular. Despite the lack of visuals, that does not mean that this category of experience is any less intense than its counterparts.

Patients undergoing an energetic experience will begin to feel large amounts of energy coursing through their body. There is no universal directionality when it comes to which way the energy flows. It often starts at the crown and moves its way down to the feet, but it may move from the feet up, or flow sideways through the body.

The patient may begin to feel painful memories or traumas that have been locked up in the body begin to be shaken loose by the energies flowing through them. When this happens, they will experience intense emotions. For example, if someone almost got into a car accident while in traffic, but never took the time to breathe through the experience because they were in a rush to get to work, that experience gets locked away in the subconscious. In this kind of experience, it will reemerge, and the patient will re-experience all of the emotions of the moment flowing through the body.

The patient may feel an overpowering desire to shake, vibrate, rock, or otherwise engage in fast, repetitive motions. This movement is a way that the nervous system is processing the trauma, literally working to "shake it off", and send it out of the physical body. If this happens, do not fight it by trying to remain still. The patient should not be worried about disturbing others near them; the shaman will ensure the process goes smoothly. Patients may also become sensitive to the energies of other patients' energies in the maloca.

Insightful:

Some experiences with ayahuasca can be very difficult. The patient may have to feel as if they are slogging through mud in order to make it through the experience. Other varieties can be breathtaking in their simplicity. This may be the case with some insightful experiences.

When it comes to this variety of experience, there is usually a problem that has been vexing the patient, either consciously or unconsciously. The aspect of the patient's life that needs healing may be something they had not paid attention to, had not previously considered or had not wanted to consider. The medicine takes the opportunity of the ceremony to shine a bright spotlight on these areas.

This may come across as a sudden understanding, or a flash of insight into the mind of the patient. It may feel as if a blurry picture snapped into focus, or as if many jumbled puzzle pieces fell into place. Whatever the problem that is making the patient's life more difficult is (a lack of money, a chronic illness, etc.) this kind of experience gives a sudden jolt of understanding as to the root cause. It should be noted, however, that learning the root cause may be a jarring and unpleasant experience. After all, it is never pleasant to learn that one's difficulties are one's own fault, whether through direct action or neglect.

In the process of revealing the root cause of an issue, the spirit of ayahuasca may bring forgotten things to the surface. This may take the form of the patient remembering an action they had taken some time ago, or a set of seemingly unimportant, unrelated circumstances. The patient may even begin to remember people from long ago in their past, perhaps classmates that they went to kindergarten with. As the patient remembers these things, connections and insights may emerge naturally, like cream rising to the top of milk—or it may emerge suddenly, like a strike of lighting.

Purgative:

Perhaps one of the most harrowing varieties of experience is someone can experience under the influence of the medicine is the purgative experience. This experience may be accompanied by images, or it may not have a visionary component at all.

The patient may feel as if there is a feeling of denseness lodged somewhere in their physical body. It may be located in their intestines, stomach muscles, or spine (etc.). Once the purge begins, the act of vomiting may feel as if it is dislodging these dense energies from their harborages. They are literally getting "shaken up," and then symbolically and/or literally purged through the vomit.

As this is happening, the patient may get the distinct impression that they are releasing traumas and old ingrained patterns through whatever orifice they happen to be purged from the most powerful purgative experiences tend to coincide with vomit. People undergoing this kind of experience describe it as joyous and liberating; thought it may seem an issue of cognitive dissonance to attribute joy with the act of vomiting, it does occur.

Some people have even been reported to laugh or cry with relief as they are vomiting. The physical act of vomiting is a potent means for energetic, mental, and emotional purge. It is an excellent, and often joyous, experience for one to let go of something that they have carried for so long. People carry burdens through their lives for decades. A woman may hold onto guilt or shame over hurting a friend over thirty years ago. A man may hold onto regret at leaving a friend in their time of need. Someone may hold onto anger at an employer who wronged them many years ago. Being invited to set these burdens down is one of the greatest gifts that ayahuasca can give to a patient. They may feel "hollowed out," and clearer than they have in decades.

Traumatic:

There are many people who have an amazing experience under the influence of ayahuasca. They may experience radical self-forgiveness, put down burdens they have carried for decades, or they may confront their most deeply repressed traumas. There is another kind of experience that is not often talked about, though. This experience usually entails a disorienting and unprecedented surge of emotion that comes seemingly out of nowhere. The patient may leave the ceremony feeling disoriented and disturbed.

These kinds of experiences may occur when the body is seeking to release traumas that were repressed while the patient was still a pre-verbal child. When people are infants, they are too young to have any resiliency to process trauma. The only way to survive mentally intact is for the body and mind to repress the trauma. When these traumas emerge, they come from nowhere. Just as the infant mind is unable to make sense of the trauma when it is happening, the ayahuasca experience may be experiencing, overwhelming, and lacking any kind of logic or meaning.

The key to dealing with this kind of experience is to let it flow through. The body is attempting to process a trauma long forgotten. It is like a storm; it rises up, and all that the patient can do is ride it out and wait for it to subside. Once the clouds have blown past, the body will have processed and released the repressed trauma. However, the experience may leave the patient feeling shaken and unsteady.

While integration is vital to any ayahuasca experience, it is even more important when people undergo this kind of experience. If they do not have proper assistance to help them "land" back into daily reality, an experience of this intensity can leave them vulnerable and unmoored. Ensuring proper support after the experience will help the patient regain their equilibrium after a dramatic and scary experience.

Initiatory:

Some experiences while under the influence of ayahuasca have an initiatory quality. The way that the initiation manifests varies from person to person, but the experience itself is usually a harrowing one. There is usually some quality of experience death, or walking through deep and terrifying darkness. The initiation occurs once the patient has made it through the darkness.

The patient may find themselves confronted by spirits associated with ayahuasca. The spirits that conduct initiation tend to be the more imposing variety, commonly in the form of a jaguar or giant anaconda. Patients may find themselves confronting the open mouth of the spirit, and find themselves swallowed whole.

Patients may also find themselves dismembered at the hands of the spirits, either at the claws of the jaguar or torn apart by small demons or other beings. The experience of having one's flesh rent apart is common in shamanic cultures across the world, as is being swallowed by the spirits. Either way, the patient faces their own death and the dissolution of their form into the greater whole.

They may feel the physical pain of their body being rent apart, as well as the visceral terror of facing the maw of a giant serpent. Alternatively, the patient may find themselves transported into the midst of a hellish dimension, being forced to walk through grotesqueness and suffering.

All of these experiences force the patient to abandon all previous conceptions of self. The patient must literally walk through hell, or face their death. Once they have come through the other side of these experiences, the previous version of themselves has died. The person who emerges from it is reborn and has been initiated at the hands of the spirits.

Exactly what the person has been initiated into is intensely private and individual. They may simply have been initiated into a new phase of their life, or they may have been initiated into a working relationship with a specific spirit or medicine.

Ayahuasca has a myriad of effects which are psychological, visual, and otherwise. The shaman uses a variety of techniques and tools to ensure that the experience moves forward in ways that are safe and productive. The ayahuasca experience can take many forms. It is unique to each patient, and the healing that is received may look very different from person to person. No matter what it looks like, it is a potent opportunity for the patient to address some of their darkest shadows.

CHAPTER 6
Long-Term Effects

The previous chapters have led the reader through the various steps up to, and into, the ayahuasca experience. This chapter will address what happens after. There are many things that need consideration. The patient's work is not done just because the ceremony has come to an end. The after-effects of ayahuasca are just as, if not more important, than the ceremonial experience. The below sections will touch on the importance of integration, and the long-term psychological effects and benefits in regards to numerous mental health conditions such as addiction and PTSD.

The Importance of Integration

One thing that most people don't realize about experiencing ayahuasca is that the experience with the plant medicine doesn't end just because the ceremony is over. The plant's insights and even spirit may remain with a person for weeks or months after the ceremony.

The ceremony itself can be considered akin to getting open-heart surgery at the hands of the plant medicine. The person has been opened up, shaken, and expunged and purged dense energies. Just as it takes time to heal from surgery, it takes time to return to equilibrium after drinking ayahuasca. The time necessary for integration is a small price to pay to ensure the patient does not regress or backslide.

After someone has surgery to get their appendix removed, they're not getting up and trying to go to work the next day. They understand that the physical body needs time to stitch itself back together and heal. Ayahuasca does something equivalent to the mind.

Dietary Recommendations

When healing from spiritual surgery—as one might think of an ayahuasca experience—nourishment is very important. Taking care of the body is akin to taking care of the mind and the spirit. The patient who is integrating after an ayahuasca experience should make sure they are eating whole, healthful foods to support their healing process.

The patient should do their best to avoid foods that are highly processed and high in refined sugars and salt. The time after the ceremony is an important time for the patient to flex their willpower to stay the course. If the patient finds themselves backsliding into unhealthy eating habits, it can quickly evolve into regression on other unhealthy or addictive patterns of behavior

This is also an excellent opportunity for the patient to pick up new, healthier habits—including eating habits. Due to the way ayahuasca works, it promotes neuroplasticity. The brain is able to forge new connections and pick up new patterns. There is a good chance that new habits picked up now will stick.

Daily Practice

Picking up a daily mindfulness practice is a great way to help the patient integrate their experience. Meditation is one such mindfulness practice. Meditation helps the adherent to tame their thoughts, and to create a more peaceful mind. Being able to create space and quiet in the mind is vital in order to do the work of self-examination that comes after ayahuasca. It allows one to cultivate a sense of strength and bravery in facing the self.

Journaling is another excellent way to integrate after an ayahuasca experience. The thoughts can get jumbled and messy throughout the day. Taking the time to order them out on paper can be likened to straightening out one's thoughts inside one's own mind. Writing something down can help someone figure out how they feel about it, and what their true feelings are. Writing can help one sense larger patterns emerging from their thoughts, and go even deeper into their healing.

Finding Community

Finding a group or community to help one through the integration process is also a wonderful idea. Ideally, one would have a support network already in place prior to the ayahuasca experience, so that they could rely on that network once they return.

Finding a community is recommended, quite simply, because it is extremely different to go it alone. Bearing the weight of self-examination and spiritual surgery can be too much for someone to deal with by themselves. Being able to share the experience with trusted friends, family or community can greatly aid in the healing process. Humans are social creatures; they are not meant to stay silent and alone.

Besides this, people often learn the deepest truths about themselves once they see that truth reflected in another person. The patient may learn a deep-seated truth about their own healing by seeing themselves reflected in a trusted friend or family member. In this way, the community greatly speeds and streamlines the healing process.

Spending Time in Nature

It is also a good idea for the patient to make time to escape into nature periodically after their ayahuasca experience. The hectic nature of modern life, especially in large cities, can take up a lot of mental space. The busyness of outer life translates into the busyness of the mind, making it hard for the patient to find the mental time and space to do any integration.

Aside from making space in the mind, getting out into nature can also help the patient get back into touch with the sacred, in the form of the plant spirits. They may be able to rekindle the transformative power that was awakened the night of the ceremony.

Being away from the hectic nature of modernity also gives the patient a chance to re-ground themselves. That grounded space allows the spirits of the plants to continue to speak to the patient. If the patient's mind is busy and clouded, and they are far away from nature, the plant spirits will not be able to communicate effectively.

Exercise the Body

Neuroplasticity is a wonderful thing; it allows the patient the opportunity to pick up new habits with the potential to become lasting. One of the habits it is recommended that the patient pick up is some kind of physical practice to tone and strengthen the body.

During the ayahuasca experience, traumas that were locked up in the body were released and expunged. Now that those things have been forcibly removed, there is a new space in the body. That space creates the potential for greater health and well-being. If the patient taps into that potential, they can reach new heights of health and wellbeing.

On the opposite side, if the patient ignores this opportunity, they may find themselves regressing. Ayahuasca gives the patient a great gift, in the form of many opportunities to grow, change, and improve. If the patient squanders that opportunity, they may find themselves worse off than when they started.

Long-term Psychological Benefits

The previous section detailed the importance of integration and provided some advice and methods for patients to follow. The people who have the most successful experiences and lasting change from working with ayahuasca are the ones who take time to integrate. The following sections will outline the benefits that ayahuasca provides to people with a wide variety of mental illnesses, including PTSD, depression, addiction, and anxiety.

Addiction

Ayahuasca is an excellent treatment for people who suffer from addiction. Purists who adhere to systems such as AA believe that it is impossible to treat one drug addiction by providing another drug. They are sadly misguided.

The reason that ayahuasca is such an effective treatment for addiction is that addiction is a coping mechanism and a signal for unprocessed trauma. There are many varieties of addiction, not just limited to drugs. People can be addicted to nearly anything. Aside from being addicted to drugs, people can be addicted to physical things, such as food. People develop addictions to sex, gambling, pornography, masturbation, and the internet. People may also find themselves with a criminal addiction, such as kleptomania or pyromania—the addiction to setting fires.

Why do these addictions manifest? Addiction is, in its simplest terms, a coping mechanism. There is some pain or wound in the subconscious mind that is so crippling that a bizarre and unhealthy set of behaviors sprouted up in order to help the conscious mind cope with it. The pain or wound is usually acquired at some point in early childhood. Many people who have addictive personalities did not have their needs met as a child for love or stability. They may also have suffered abuse—verbal, physical, or sexual—at the hands of someone who was supposed to be trusted. The trauma is also occasionally acquired later in life, with addictive symptoms not manifesting until later.

The trauma is not able to be fully repressed. Thus, the body and brain figure out workarounds to help the body cope with the trauma. In order to prevent the conscious mind from drowning in darkness and despair constantly, the mind figures out external sources to activate the reward centers in the brain. The addictive behavior allows the person to experience hits of dopamine that makes them feel good and keep them moving and able to get through their day.

Of course, this survival strategy is ultimately destructive and may be deadly. Ayahuasca is so helpful because it helps people to tackle their addiction at the source, which is the trauma that caused the addictive behavior to evolve in the first place.

There are many reasons that ayahuasca succeeds in treating addiction where other methods fail. One of these reasons is that it does not require talking. Methods such as talk therapy can be excruciating for people who have difficulty opening up to other people. Finding the words to articulate one's inner pain can be an insurmountable task for many of those suffering from addiction. Ayahuasca takes the healing conversation directly into the mind of the patient, freeing the patient from the anxiety of having to talk to a psychiatrist.

Another reason that ayahuasca is so useful in treating addiction is that it not only provides healing to the mind but also improves the health of the physical structures of the brain. The medicine can boost the health of areas of the brain such as the insula and amygdala. The period of neuroplasticity that ayahuasca provides after the experience also allows new neural connections and pathways to be formed. These new pathways are physically "rewiring" the brain to help it heal from the trauma that caused the addiction.

Aside from the benefits to the purely physical structures of the brain, the medicine also heals the mind and thought patterns. People who undergo an experience with the medicine report an increased degree of insight into their own history and the root causes of their addiction. They also report an increased reflective capacity, or a greater ability to look back at their history and thoughts and recognize patterns. Not only this, but they are better able to think critically about the sources of their trauma, and to decide upon new patterns of behavior that they wish to implement.

Ayahuasca's ability to literally rewire the brain allows people to take on completely new mindsets. People have reported their perspectives undergoing fundamental shifts. After drinking ayahuasca, people who were close-minded and resistant to change have opened up and become much more flexible in their opinions and willingness to evolve and grow. On a physical level, this can be linked to how the ayahuasca experience allows communication between parts of the brain that do not normally connect. Bridging these connections opens people up to completely new worldviews. This is especially useful for people suffering from addiction, allowing them to face hard truths and truly perceive the root of their trauma.

Several scientific studies have been conducted to investigate and quantify the effects of ayahuasca on patients. One of these studies followed addicts for several months after their ayahuasca ceremonies. They measured an overall decline in addictive drug usage. The metrics of decline included decreased usage of alcohol, tobacco, and cocaine. Patients were successfully able to implement impulse control.

There was also no observable indication that the ayahuasca had any negative effect on the patients whatsoever. While shamans throughout the Amazon know this to be fact, it has taken Western medicine a moment to catch up. A properly-conducted ayahuasca ceremony with proper integration afterwards will have no harmful effects on the patient. Aside from there being no observable harm, as well as reduced drug usage, patients also reported a greater degree of understanding and improved capacity for self-reflection. Patients were better able to understand the reasons behind their addiction. They were able to identify they traumas that they were using the addiction to medicate against.

Patients were better able to engage in problem-solving around their addictive behaviors. They were capable of identifying triggers for cravings, and understanding how the trigger and the craving were related. Not only this, but they also managed to alter their behaviors in order to productively manage the cravings without indulging it.

Finally, the patients experienced a drastic reduction in the actual number of cravings experienced. More than 50% of patients tracked reported a reduction in cravings after the ayahuasca experience. The patients not only gained a better understanding of the traumas at the roots of their addiction, but they were also better able to manage their cravings and problem-solve around them and experienced a reduction in the number of cravings overall.

PTSD

Another debilitating mental illness that is greatly alleviated by ayahuasca is PTSD. This ailment of the mind arises when one experiences a traumatic event in their life. This event overwhelms the conscious mind; the mind is unable to process it. In order to avoid being completely shattered by the event, the consciousness subsumes the event into the subconscious mind, where it waits, repressed. Though repressed, external triggers can cause flare-ups and force the patient to relive the event. These episodes are debilitating and overwhelming to the sufferer. Post-Traumatic Stress Disorder, especially the variety that is combat-related, is notoriously resistant to treatment. Ayahuasca works as a form of assisted exposure therapy. When people who have experienced trauma avoid situations that induce fear, it does nothing to help them heal; rather, it only maintains and reinforces the deep, ingrained conditioning underlying their illness.

By digging up traumatic memories and exposing the conscious mind to them in a controlled, safe environment, the medicine provides the brain with a unique opportunity to reassess and, hopefully, extinguish fear responses that have been conditioned into the mind. This allows people a method to access the trauma that prevents them from being overwhelmed by it and to address the fear around the trauma.

On a purely chemical level, ayahuasca modulates activity in the brain, gene expression, epigenetic regulation, and neurotransmission. The DMT component of ayahuasca activates SIGMAR1, the sigma 1 receptor, among others. SIGMAR1 has many jobs, being a stress-responsive receptor site. It has a hand in many areas, such as cell survival, protection, and plasticity of neurons, and others. Traumatic memories are often repressed, and patients who take ayahuasca report the reemergence of these memories.

This can be linked to the SIGMAR1 receptor site being activated by the DMT contained in ayahuasca. Ayahuasca hyper-activates the SIGMAR1 receptor site and brings the memories forward. Once the memories are brought forward, they become destabilized and malleable. Ayahuasca, with the ability to promote neurogenesis and neuroplasticity, can help to reform the memory.

The medicine works by boosting the processes involved with the reconsolidation of memories and the extinction of fear. Thus, when the memory arises, it can be effectively reprogrammed, and the fear it sparks can be extinguished. The reprogrammed memory is then stored in the consciousness so that the memory will no longer trigger the patient.

Now that the biological mechanisms underlying the effects of ayahuasca on PTSD have been outlined, it is expedient to delineate how this chemistry plays out in the brain as a visionary experience. The mental and psychological experience of patients is highly variable and subjective, but there are a few commonalities across the range of experiences.

The most common occurrence is for the patient to feel as if they are reliving the experience. This occurs in one of two ways. In the first variety, they may experience a replaying of the event on a kind of mental "television screen," observing the events as they unfold. In the second variety, the patient may experience a kind of time distortion, and feel as if the past and the present are co-occuring simultaneously. They may relieve the event as if it is taking place in that very moment, surrounded by all of the sensory information and input in the moment of the traumatic event.

However, when the traumatic event resurfaces, it does not re-traumatize the patient as it did in the original moment. Instead, as mentioned in the previous paragraphs, ayahuasca allows the patient's brain an opportunity to reassess the threat from the memory, and to re-tag the memory. The repeated exposure to the trauma serves as exposure therapy, lessening the shock of the memory through repeated witnessing. The ability to rewatch or re-experience the trauma allows the mind to divorce the trauma from the ingrained fear response, recoding the memory so that it no longer serves as a trigger for PTSD episodes.

Once the memory has been brought up to the surface and processed by the brain, it is the mental and emotional equivalent of receiving open heart surgery. Just as with major surgery, aftercare is vitally important. A patient is not sent home the day after having their aorta operated on; just so, a patient that is processing memories associated with PTSD must take extreme diligence with aftercare protocols.

If those protocols are followed correctly, amazing things can result. A documentary, *From Shock to Awe*, followed a group of veterans who were all individually coping with combat-related PTSD. The documentary and descriptive, and was more interested in the subjective markers of well-being and improvement in each of the veterans, rather than in attempting to quantify the result.

At the end of the documentary, many of the veterans in the film found immense relief from the symptoms of their PTSD. Not only did they find relief from their acute symptoms, but they also were able to process the traumatic event that dwelled at the root of their disorder. Veterans who were previously barely able to perform basic tasks such as running to the grocery store found themselves transformed and healed.

It is a well-known fact that the treatment options for American veterans are woefully underequipped. In many cases, traditional treatment methods can actually cause the symptoms of PTSD to worsen, leaving the patient unable to function and perform day to day tasks.

The ayahuasca, especially the purgative aspect of the plant, allows sufferers of PTSD a chance to let go of the damaged parts of themselves. Many patients have reported feeling as if they were vomiting out their memories, and felt the death of the self that was broken. The new self, with a healed mind, is able to step forward into their life unburdened of the trauma that has haunted their conscious and subconscious minds.

The complex chemical processes bring about powerful and transformative psychological and visionary experiences that allow the patient the opportunity to bring the trauma to the surface in a safe and controlled way. In this space, they can recondition their brain's reaction to the memory, and extinguish their fear once and for all.

Depression

Depression is an extremely complex disease, and the exact origin has yet to be pinned down by modern medicine. On its most basic level, depression is caused by lower than normal amounts of neurotransmitters in the brain. These three neurotransmitters are dopamine, serotonin, and norepinephrine. Scientists are unsure why these neurotransmitters are in low supply in the first place. It is possible that the body simply does not produce enough of them, that there aren't enough receptor sites to receive them, or that the enzymes and molecules necessary to produce them simply aren't present.

The symptoms that result from the shortage of these neurotransmitters are nothing short of catastrophic. They may be as "mild" as simply being unable to find the motivation to shower or get out of bed. In their most extreme cases, it can lead to suicidal ideation as a hope for release from the pain of this disorder.

On a purely chemical level, ayahuasca works by sending DMT to the serotonin receptor sites in the brain. Once DMT has entered the receptor site, the brain begins to be flooded with serotonin. This "flooding" effect can perhaps be one reason that people who suffer from depression—and thus, have lower than normal levels of serotonin and other neurotransmitters in their brain—feel such relief after an ayahuasca ceremony.

Due to the complexity of the disorder of depression, it is difficult to pinpoint exactly how the biochemical components of ayahuasca alleviate the symptoms of depression in relation to the patient's neurochemistry. However, as anyone should well know by this point, the benefits of ayahuasca transcend the purely chemical and take up their highest degree of healing in the realm of the spiritual.

That spiritual dynamic is precisely where the most dramatic healing occurs. People who suffer from depression will experience a resurfacing of long-forgotten traumas, as well as negative patterns of behavior that contribute to the disease in their overall mental health. This is typically where the "insightful" category of ayahuasca experience comes into play, revealing to the patient the roots of their disorders and disease.

During the ayahuasca experience, patients who suffer from depression may have an intense experience of "coming alive" or "jolting awake" after having spent a long time half-asleep. They may experience repressed emotions intensely or experience a breakthrough sense of long-forgotten wonder and awe at the mysteries of the universe. However it manifests, there is the sense of the emotions "waking up," allowing the patient to feel emotions intensely for the first time in months or years.

Ideally, someone would dive deeply into the source of their trauma and begin to address the root causes of their mental health challenges. Some do not. Even for those who do not put in the work, they will typically see an alleviation of the symptoms of depression for approximately three months afterward. After the three-month threshold has been reached, they may have to re-dose.

For those who do begin to do the work of addressing their trauma, the effects may be more long-lasting. However, the task of processing trauma is work that must be carried out over months or years. Repeated doses are usually necessary. However, if someone is dedicated to doing the work, they may find permanent healing.

Anxiety Disorders

There are several kinds of anxiety disorder. The first kind is a panic disorder, which causes panic attacks with no discernable external stimulus. The second kind is a social anxiety disorder, which causes a debilitating stress reaction to everyday interpersonal interactions. Generalized anxiety disorder refers to strong anxiety and stress response to everyday stimuli. Finally, specific phobias also fall under the category of anxiety disorder.

Anxiety disorders are caused by chemical imbalances in the brain, just as depression is. However, the exact mechanisms that cause anxiety disorders are not fully understood by scientists at this time. Scientists have observed that being under high levels of stress for a prolonged period of time can cause someone to develop an anxiety disorder.

The symptoms of anxiety disorders include feelings of panic, uneasiness, and fear; obsessive thoughts; insomnia; repetitive behaviors; palpitations; inability to sit still; nausea, muscle tension, and numbness. When the patient drinks ayahuasca, they will experience the serotonin-flooding effects, causing parts of the brain that don't normally communicate to connect. This flood of neurotransmitter may be what is responsible for the alleviation of symptoms that many people feel after drinking ayahuasca. Sufferers of anxiety disorders often report feeling lighter, less obsessive, and less tense after drinking ayahuasca.

However, it should be noted that during the ayahuasca experience a temporary intensification of their anxiety symptoms. This is usually linked to the re-experiencing of trauma that happens to people under the influence of the medicine. It is important to note that this intensification is temporary, and a part of the "purge" that happens in relation to ayahuasca.

The patient may find themselves journeying to their distant childhood, to the traumatic events that happened that caused them to develop the trait of hyper-vigilance in the first place. Once they re-experience the trauma, it loses its grip on their mind, and they are able to move past it.

People who are able to successfully process their trauma and alleviate their anxiety demonstrate lowered levels of stress hormone in their system—an effect that can be permanent.

One study handed out surveys to people with anxiety disorders who had drunk ayahuasca. It tracked their markers of well-being for several months after the experience. Patients reported lower levels of anxiety for months after the experience, as well as lowered levels of overall stress.

Patients also reported that their satisfaction with life was significantly increased the day after the ceremony, and their self-reported markers of well-being also showed marked increases. Overall, the study demonstrated that people who ingested ayahuasca experienced significant improvement with their symptoms, at least as far as self-reporting tools can measure. At this time no study has looked into the neurochemistry of anxiety following ayahuasca sessions.

Ayahuasca is an amazing tool to treat an incredibly diverse host of mental health concerns. The experience is intense, and as such, needs to be given proper time for integration. It is the equivalent of receiving psychological surgery to release trauma. As long as the proper time for integration is allotted, the patients will most likely experience marked improvements in a huge host of areas. People suffering from PTSD reported being able to go back to the moment of trauma and purge the fear; many people no longer qualified for the PTSD label after the experience. Likewise, people with anxiety, addiction and depression have found lasting healing in the hands of the ayahuasca ceremony.

CONCLUSION

Thank you for making it through to the end of *Ayahuasca: Sacred Plant Medicine of the Amazon Jungle*. Let's hope it was informative and able to provide you with all of the tools you need to achieve your goals, whatever they may be.

The next step is to take all of the information you have learned and to decide if the ayahuasca experience is right for you. If you believe it is, then it is imperative that you get serious about your research. You will want to find a legitimate retreat center and/or ayahuasquero you wish to work with in the jungle. Once you have identified the place where you wish to partake of the medicine, you will need to pay whatever their rate is in exchange for the experience.

After you have made your reservation, it is time to ready yourself for the intense preparation regimen. You will need to abide by the strict diet and cut out all refined sugars, salts, pork, red meat, and fermented foods from your diet. Anything containing tyramine must be eliminated. You must also ensure that you are not taking any medications that are contraindicated with any component of ayahuasca, including DMT and MAOI. You will need to avoid sexual contact for at least two weeks prior. Ensure that after your experience you allot proper time and resources to your integration.

Finally, if you found this book useful in any way, a review on Amazon is always appreciated!

DESCRIPTION

Ayahuasca: Sacred Plant Medicine of the Amazon Jungle provides a quick yet comprehensive look into a topic that is often intimidating to broach. Ayahuasca is a plant medicine that has been used by Amazonian shamans for thousands of years and is surrounded by an extremely dense web of spiritual lore and cultural protocols. It can be scary to dive into this world, but the chapters of this book make the world of ayahuasca easy and accessible. It will provide you with everything the prospective psychonauts might need to know before journeying into the realm of the plant spirits. This book will:

- Give the reader a thorough understanding of the history and cultural importance of the ayahuasca plant.
- Dive deeply into the spiritual mythos surrounding ayahuasca, providing a thorough look at the different spirits associated with the plant. These include, but are not limited to: the ayahuasca plant itself, the spirit of the jaguar, and the spirit of the anaconda.
- Define the role and training of the shaman, and the rigorous training they must undergo before being permitted to administer and oversee ayahuasca experiences.
- Describe the ways in which the shaman facilitates and steers the experience, including but not limited to their use of sacred songs called *icaros*, the purifying substance is known as Florida water, and the sacred tobacco called *mapacho*.
- Outline the psychoactive components of the plant and provide a detailed account of how ayahuasca works in the body and affects brain chemistry.
- Explain which medications are contraindicated with ayahuasca, and the potential interactions and side effects that can occur if one mixes prescription drugs with the medicine.
- Provide information regarding the preparatory diet, as well as an explanation of what tyramine is, its dangerous interactions with ayahuasca, and why one must avoid eating foods that contain it
- Outline other aspects of the preparation regimen, including behavioral protocols that must be followed prior to ayahuasca ingestion. These protocols involve avoiding sexual contact of all kinds, as well as taking up a daily mindfulness practice.
- Delineate some common categories of experience people undergo after drinking the medicine of ayahuasca, and how to handle the experiences as they arise.
- Show how to successfully integrate after the experience, as well as describe the long-term benefits ayahuasca has been shown to effect in people suffering from various kinds of mental illnesses, including PTSD, depression, and addiction.

Ayahuasca: Sacred Plant Medicine of the Amazon Jungle is a one-stop shop for anything the potential journeyer might need to know about this amazing and transformative sacrament. It has been used in the jungle for countless generations, and only in modern times have Westerners been able to access this life-changing experience. With this book as your guide, you will have everything you need to know to begin planning your own experience.

CPSIA information can be obtained
at www.ICGtesting.com
Printed in the USA
BVHW060844020621
608483BV00004BA/1346